# CATARACT SURGERY AND PHACOEMULSIFICATION FOR THE BEGINNING SURGEONS

**DR.S.M.MUNIRUL HUQ**
FRCS (GLASG), DO, FRCOphth(UK)
FACS (USA)
EX PROFESSOR OF OPHTHALMOLOGY
HOLY FAMILY RED CRESCENT MEDICAL COLLEGE
DHAKA, BANGLADESH
AND
**DR. MEHDI (MATTI) VAZEEN, MD**
MEDICAL DIRECTOR
CENTER FOR ADVANCED EYE CARE
1104 N. DIVISION STREET
CARSON CITY NV 89703, USA

authorHOUSE®

AuthorHouse™
1663 Liberty Drive
Bloomington, IN 47403
www.authorhouse.com
Phone: 1-800-839-8640

Note: This book is for educational and training purposes only and is published in good faith to help the trainee doctors.

While every effort has been made by the authors to confirm the accuracy of the information contained herein to describe the surgical procedures and are presented with the experience by the authors and are in line with the generally accepted practices. However, the authors or the publishers are not responsible for any unintentional errors or omissions and are not responsible for any consequences from the application of the information contained in this book and makes no warranty, expressed or implied, in respect to the completeness of the contents of the publication. Practice and application of the information contained herein at a particular situation remains the professional responsibility of the practitioner. The drugs and devices and machinery described in this book are in accordance to the current recommendations and practice at the time of publication, but the reader is urged to check the drug or devices with the original manufactures of the drug or the device for correctness.   Whenever the reader is in doubt, the authors recommend that the original articles published on the topic should be consulted. Every effort has been made for the correctness of the contents but some unintentional errors in spelling or description may be encountered for which the authors are not responsible and express regret. The products described in the text are believed to be approved by the FDA (USA). It is the responsibility of the reader to ascertain the FDA status of the products before using them in practice. Neither the Publishers nor the Authors assumes any liability for any damage or injury and /or damage to the person or property arising out of or related to any use of the materials contained in this book. The reader may or may not use the medicines, equipments or procedures as described in this book at his or her own discretion. The reader is urged to consult a consultant, guide or mentor before performing any or all procedures described in this book. Phacoemulsification for the Beginning surgeons

Published by AuthorHouse      11/06/2014

ISBN: 978-1-4969-4413-9 (sc)
ISBN: 978-1-4969-4412-2 (e)

# DEDICATED TO

## FROM DR. HUQ
MY PARENTS, MY PATIENTS AND MY FAMILY (RITA,
NOWARA, NAVED, ZAKI AND ZAZYDEN)
### AND
# DEDICATED TO

## FROM DR. MEHDI VAZEEN
TO MY PARENTS, MY TEACHERS AND MY
FAMILY (ASHLEY, CAMERON AND BELLA)

# CONTENTS

# FOREWORD

Cataract is the leading cause of blindness in many developing countries. Many people in these countries cannot afford to have the surgery done and remain as a blind person for the rest of their lives. The enormous burden of cataract blindness cannot be met by the Government alone, or charitable organizations who are working hard in these countries to combat the malady.

Recent development in the surgical techniques, lenses and instrumentation has brought about additional burden on the ophthalmologists to learn the new techniques and be proficient.

The only way to address the problem of cataract blindness is to develop manpower so that the surgeries can be performed. The authors with their vast experience have attempted to offer guidance for the new cataract surgeons.

We have tried to keep this book simple yet relevant. The steps outlined give the new surgeons a starting point on his journey in becoming an experienced surgeon.

It has to be remembered that proficiency is gained only by repeated practice.

This book is not intended to give all the answers but it is a good beginning to lay the groundwork for a lifetime of learning and eventually leading to becoming a proficient surgeon.

The new surgeons can use this book to create the necessary steps in starting his education and training in becoming a cataract surgeon. The words in this book are from practicing surgeon's day to day experience in how to handle patient care from the time they enter the clinic to the time they have their surgery done and leave satisfied.

We hope that the trainee surgeon find these chapters to be relevant and helpful in their pursuit in becoming a good cataract surgeon.

There is no better gift or life altering experience for the surgeon when they operate on a blind person and give the gift of sight.

This will hopefully be a call to all surgeons to continually teach and train others to achieve their goal.

**Dr. Mehdi (Matti) Vazeen MD**
**Medical Director**
Center for Advanced Eye Care
1104, Division Street
Carson City, Nevada 89703, USA

## Preface

# PREFACE BY DR. S.M.MUNIRUL HUQ

Phacoemulsification or simply phaco surgery has become synonymous with cataract surgery in the present time. Two decades ago patients would come with complains of poor vision and would ask the doctor for treatment. Now the patients presents to the doctor to ask for phaco surgery with foldable lens implant. The instrumentation, technological advancements and patient education has improved during this time. More advancement is yet to come with incorporation of Laser in phaco techniques and improvement in the pump mechanisms in the machines. I have been performing cataract surgery for more than the past four decades from the age of Intracapsular Cataract Extraction to present day Phacoemulsification. This book is a true reflection of my learning curve of cataract surgery and portrays the different stages I had to go through during my lifetime. Time has changed and today with a click on U tube, one can find hundreds of videos of cataract surgeries. But just two decades ago, we had no such advantage and had to stand for hours in order to observe a live surgery. During the process of learning a new technique there is a need for training guide. Young surgeons need to learn the procedure quickly and efficiently to deliver the optimum results to their patients. The surgeon therefore must learn the surgical steps and be a master in the technique and also learn what to do when things go wrong. Thus learning how to convert to Small Incision Cataract Surgery or Extracapsular Cataract Surgery in addition to phaco surgical techniques is important. It is also important to learn what to do if there are complications. With this scenario in mind my intention to write this book is to give a practical guide to the trainee ophthalmologists. The established phaco surgeons may use this guide to teach and train students.

The book focuses upon the practical aspects of the surgery without much theoretical details. Getting used to an operating microscope is difficult for the beginners and a separate chapter deals with the technique to get adjusted to the operating microscope. The book deals with the basic description of each step associated with cataract surgery and the more the surgeons practice the steps, the more proficiency will be gained. The surgeon can then learn more sophisticated techniques. I am blessed to have a friend, Dr. Matti Vazeen MD, who is a world class experienced surgeon and he has contributed significantly in writing the book and also wrote the chapters on Refractive cataract surgery and specialty IOL implantation techniques. In fact cataract surgery has become so accurate at the present time that, with the help of appropriate instruments and skills we can reach up to 0.25 D of accuracy post operatively and even offer a better quality of vision. Pre existing astigmatism can be treated at the same time by planning the surgery and using the correction techniques. I am grateful to Dr. Matti Vazeen for writing these chapters and also for overall guidance to write the book. He has reviewed each chapter meticulously and modified the text to be more meaningful and worthwhile for the new surgeons. Dr. Karl Holzinger MD is a great friend who has supported me in writing the book and also encouraged me at every step in my life. I am indebted to him for holding my hand during my first phaco surgery and being my trainer in the first 20 phaco surgeries I performed and he travelled 16000 miles from USA to Bangladesh to do so.

I am deeply indebted to my teachers, Late Prof. Mustafizur Rahman FRCS, Late Prof. M.A. Matin FRCS, Late Prof. M.A. Jalil FRCS, Prof. Sayed Modasser Ali FRCS, Dr. M.R Nanjiani FRCS, Dr. J.C.Chawla FRCS, and Prof. Gordon Dutton FRCS to train me in Ophthalmology and supporting me throughout my career. I am extremely grateful to Prof. W.S.Foulds FRCS, Past President of the Royal College of Ophthalmologists, UK for his support during my study in U.K. I shall fail my duties if I do not express my gratitude to Mr. Christopher E.B. Friend and Mr. Abu Baker Siddique of Sight Savers UK, for the support they have extended during my training in UK. I am very indebted that Late Mr. Alan Jones and Mr. Kevin Kerry of Sight Savers, UK had faith in me and offered me the opportunities at the right time to get myself trained and qualified to be an ophthalmologist.

This book could not be written without the help and encouragement of many of my friends, colleagues and my family. My mother Sajeda Khanam was a source of guidance and she used to guide through endless stories of every topic of life situation. Her courage and sacrifice was the main reason that I could go to Medical School from a remote township and fulfill her dreams. My brother, Bashirul Huq has encouraged me to write and so is my sister, Nahaz Fatema. My wife Jesmine Huq (Rita) has helped me at every step of my life and I am deeply indebted to her for her love, understanding and encouragement throughout my life. If it would not be her support, I would not be what I am today and I must acknowledge that I owe her for all the good and wonderful things that life has given me. I am grateful to God for making all my endeavors in life successful. My daughter, Nowara Munir is a breeze of fresh air in my life. She is a constant source of love, encouragement and enthusiasm for whatever my wish lists are from sightseeing, traveling, going to concerts to writing a book. I feel greatly satisfied that my son, Naved Munir has chosen to be a doctor. He has read and criticized some of the chapters and I had rewritten them. He is very understanding and caring for all my works and unconditionally admires me and all that I do. New addition to my life is my son in law, Zaki Choudhury who never gets tired in criticizing me but his eyes tell me how much he loves me, and my Grand Son, Zayden who is a cute little adorable baby and the best gift of God one can have. Another addition in my life is Jannat Akhter Mou who brings a breeze of heaven to my mind. Encouragement, support and love of all of these people are a constant source of enthusiasm in my life.

I must acknowledge the contribution of Prof. Muniruzzaman Bhuyan D.C.H., MBBS, PhD, Pediatrician and Principal, Holy Family Red Crescent Medical College, Dhaka for his support. He has gracefully contributed in my life and in my teaching career. He is a born leader and organizer and has organized the Holy Family Red Crescent Medical College to be one of the best Medical Colleges in the country. I am deeply indebted and grateful to him.

Finally, I must thank Dr. Mehdi (Matti)Vazeen and his wife Ashley for their support during production of the manuscript and for publication of this book. Dr. Matti is a friend who never fails and has patiently listened to my aspirations, understood them and helped me to execute my endeavors. He has rewritten each chapter to make it more useful for the beginner surgeons. It is because of their generosity that this book comes free of charge for the trainee ophthalmologists in Bangladesh and at a small cost to the ophthalmologists around the globe.

In spite of our all out efforts, we could not incorporate too many illustrations in the book. In the present day situation, plenty of videos and pictures of cataract surgery can be seen from the internet and I encourage the surgeons to use this facility so freely available to the new surgeons in order to understand the surgical steps. I want to thank Mr. Rezaul Hoque Liton, commercial artist for the illustrations and I thank Dr. Matti Vazeen and Dr Karl Holzinger for providing the pictures of their surgical steps.

There are some unintentional mistakes in the book for which I apologize. We look forward to comments and suggestions from readers for improvements. We hope that this book will be helpful for the young Ophthalmologists to learn cataract and Phaco surgery and become successful cataract surgeons.

Finally, I am deeply indebted to the publishers of this book and the printers who have spent long hours to publish this work and distribute the same.

**DR.S.M.MUNIRUL HUQ**
**FRCS, DO, FRCOPHTH, FACS**
**Ex. Professor of Ophthalmology,**
**Holy Family Red Crescent Medical College,**
**Dhaka, Bangladesh**

# Preface
# BY DR. MEHDI (MATTI) VAZEEN, M.D.

As a busy practicing cataract surgeon in Carson City, Nevada, I have been performing roughly 25 cataract surgeries every Tuesday morning for the past 18 years. I have over the years performed over 20,000 surgeries and gained some knowledge and experience with the art of performing cataract surgery.

So when my friend, Dr. Huq suggested we write a book together to help young and existing cataract surgeons in developing countries, I jumped to the idea.

I met Dr. Huq about five years ago while I was performing fifty charitable cataract surgeries in Dhaka, Bangladesh at his center. At that time I realized along with Dr. Huq the real solution to reducing over one and half million blind people in just Bangladesh is to train excellent surgeons who then can do more surgery, but more importantly, train excellent surgeons themselves.

The biggest obstacle that I have witnessed in developing countries is <u>training</u>. What I saw during my visit to Bangladesh was that the training centers are limited and there is not enough man hours available to the mentors to train new surgeons. It is important to make a conscious effort for an experienced and proficient phaco surgeon to try to help new surgeons in the skills that he has learned.

So as this book comes free for the trainee and new surgeons in Bangladesh with the cost and the time being covered by myself and Dr. Huq, I would like everyone who reads the pages in this book to promise to learn from our experiences, but more importantly, when they become masters, to help teach and train more surgeons to perform this simple and excellent procedure to new surgeons with the goal of eventually eradicating blindness due to cataracts in all the developing countries. This book will also be available for a small cost around the globe for the trainee surgeons and teaching institutions.

All surgeons who read these pages are encouraged to pay this debt forward and to train and teach any student or surgeon that is willing to learn.

I hope Dr, Huq's hard work and dedication to bring this book to new trainees and surgeons spark a change in attitude that creates a tidal wave of new surgeons teaching more surgeons once they have become the mentor.

Finally I would like to thank all my teachers at Northwestern University Medical School and Ochsner – LSU residency program especially Dr. Hesse Past Chairman, that gave me the chance and privilege to become an ophthalmologist. Their kindness and dedication has allowed me to pay it forward. We all need strong family members to support us so that we can shine. My mother and father pushed and prodded and helped me along the way. My wife Ashley, who has followed me and supported me for 18 years, and my children that give me hope have all contributed to my success and ability to write this book.

To new training surgeons, do not be afraid to push forward and become the new master to teach those that shall come after you.

God's blessing on our journey.

Mehdi (Matti) Vazeen, M.D.
**Medical Director**
**Center for Advanced Eye Care**
**1104, Division Street**
**Carson City, Nevada 89703, USA**

# Chapter 1
# INTRODUCTION

Cataract surgery is a major area of interest in Ophthalmology and great advancements has taken place in this sector during the past four decades.

In the context of the developing countries, it is very important for the ophthalmologist to learn Cataract Surgery because the number of people suffering from this disease is overwhelming. Cataract is the one of the leading causes of Blindness in Bangladesh. According to WHO estimate, there are about one and a half Million people that are blind from cataract in the country and about one hundred thousand new cases are added to this backlog per year. Naturally, a substantial portion of the clinical life of an Ophthalmologist in Bangladesh is spent to perform Cataract surgery and in management of the Patients with this disease. The same situation is prevalent in other developing countries in the world.

Approximately 48% of world blindness is due to Cataract, thus about 18 million people are blind due to cataract globally. Cataract causes moderate to severe disability in 53.8 million people in the world, (WHO estimate). In many countries, the number of cataract surgeons who can perform the surgery is limited and thus cataract remains the leading cause of blindness in the developing countries all over the world. Cataract is also an important cause of low vision in both developed and developing countries.

During my long career in Cataract Surgery, I had learned the different techniques often with extreme difficulties and hard work, and I realize and acknowledge the effort one has to go through during the learning phase of different stages of Cataract Surgery. For a beginner surgeon, it is an extremely difficult task to pursue the interest and keep on struggling to get perfection in the technique through long hours of hard work, practice and keen interest.

I have learned and convinced myself that creating trained manpower is the most important step to try to solve the problem of Cataract Blindness in the world.

There are many training and teaching hospitals in our country and in neighboring countries who are dedicatedly training Ophthalmologists to perform cataract surgery. We need more Surgeons to be trained and I believe, once a surgeon is trained, he or she will perform Cataract Surgery at any facility and they will create facilities at his or her own initiative to perform cataract surgery. The only way to combat the problem of blindness in our country and in other developing countries is to create enough trained manpower that can treat this disease.

From the very beginning of my career, I wanted to teach and train surgeons in the technique I could perform, the knowledge I had acquired with so much effort and hard work. The idea to write a book on phaco surgery based on my personal experience came to my mind logically to help the trainee surgeons. The techniques described in the book are standard procedures and every phaco surgeon performs the surgery in the same way, I am no different. The reason to write this book is to give guidance to the new surgeons how to proceed to learn Cataract surgery, be proficient in the procedure and confidently perform the surgery to deliver the best result to the patients. It is not a difficult surgery at all, but requires a lot of practice to perform every step accurately and precisely up to millimeter accuracy. This is also a guide to pre training Ophthalmologist who is eagerly trying to learn Ophthalmology and cataract surgery.

Through this book we wanted to relate our experiences and the technological details of the procedures with the trainee surgeons. The advanced Refractive Cataract Surgery has been written by an expert in this field, Dr. Mehdi Vazeen, MD. These chapters are a jewel in the book and the surgeons will be able to understand the importance of new techniques to deliver precise results. Dr. Mehdi Vazeen MD is an Ophthalmologist in USA who has performed well over 20,000 Phaco surgeries and is very proficient in the advanced techniques. He has guided me throughout the book and we have jointly reviewed the topics to make it useful and easy for the beginner surgeons. He has advised me to include topics from his vast experience and I am blessed to get his support while planning, writing and publication of this book.

During the last five decades, phacoemulsification has been a major area of interest in Ophthalmology and is one of the most rapidly developing sector of medical science with technical and instrumentation developments and advancement of knowledge. The techniques of cataract surgery has evolved from Intracapsular Cataract extraction with Capsule Forceps or Cryo machine with no lens implant and the large wound closed with four 8/0 virgin silk sutures to sutureless surgery today. Implantation of an Anterior Chamber Intraocular lens came along for a short time but went off very rapidly. Then came a decade of Extra capsular Cataract Extraction with PMMA Intraocular Lens Implant with stitches to secure the wound and next decade came with Phacoemulsification with development of Foldable Intraocular Lenses with no stitch. Simultaneously another technique of cataract surgery which gained popularity is small Incision

Cataract Surgery, SICS in our subcontinent to supplement sutureless manual cataract surgery, where Phaco machine would not be available.

This progress has not been easy for the researchers and the pioneers. All these happened as we progressed through learning curve on the different procedures of cataract surgery. Sir Harold Ridley while treating British Air force pilots injured in combat during the World War noticed that the broken PMMA pieces entering the eyes of these patients did not cause much inflammation and thought of producing a lens from this material to implant into the eye after removal of cataract. The problem of grinding the power and sterilization had to be addressed. He teamed up with Mr. John Pike Optical specialist who helped him to initially grind power into these lenses and produce an implantable design. Sir Ridley had to go through a lot of obstacles and harsh criticism while performing the initial implantations. On 29th November 1949, at St Thomas' Hospital, London, Ridley performed the first IOL operation on the eye of a 45-year-old female patient. He presented his first paper on 'Intra-Ocular Acrylic Lenses' at the Oxford Ophthalmological Congress on 9 July 1951. Anticipating criticism, Ridley had performed his early series of operations quietly and without publicity. He had implanted only three lenses in 1950 and in the same year he overcame the early problem of the calculation of the implant power.

Opposition, in the form of outright hostility, began at the Oxford presentation when several senior professional colleagues, who were to support Ridley, refused to examine two patients he had brought to the Congress. A year later in October 1952, at the American Academy meeting in Chicago, Ridley's work, in spite of his demonstration of good results, was condemned as reckless. It was not until 1981 that FDA of USA approved IOL implantation.

During the decade in 1960s, two lens designs were developed the Choyce MKVIII anterior chamber design of Peter Choyce and the 4-loop Iris Fixation lens of Cornelius Binkhorst. It was not until 1975 that John Pearce developed the first of the modern posterior chamber lens designs. This was a tripod rigid lens, but when implanted into the posterior chamber, used to sit properly centered. I had later implanted these lenses in 1984. The lens design and material changed over the next decade to the development of different PMMA designs and later, Foldable Intraocular lenses. Silicon as a foldable material came first in manufacturing foldable Intraocular lenses and to be replaced by Acrylic materials both Hydrophilic and Hydrophobic in multi piece and later single piece design, which can be implanted through small incisions.

While these revolutions in the Intraocular Lens manufacturing were going on, in 1960s, Dr. Charles Kelman MD in USA was experimenting with the possibility of removing the cataractous lens through a small incision. He was working with a research grant from John A. Hartford Foundation. His initial attempts were with a butterfly net to trap and deliver the lens, next he tried with a electric drill and a device similar to a food blender, but none of these worked because, these caused scattering of the lens fragments and damage to the cornea. He did not use these devices on human eyes. Finally, while visiting his dentist, he got the concept of developing an ultrasound device to emulsify the nucleus. Quickly, the special ultrasonic probe oscillating at 40 HZ and aspiration system were devised and by 1970, the first Kelman-Cavitron phacoemulsification machine was available. Scientists, computer experts, medical engineers and several other experts combined their efforts to bring the wonderful phacoemulsification system that we work with today. Subsequent development of phaco techniques had been a continuous modification and modernization of the different steps of the surgical technique by excellent surgeons. These advancements are well documented and will be discussed in the relevant chapters.

The journey to present day cataract surgery was not simple. It will be hard to for a surgeon today operating with the Microscope, sitting comfortably at a stool and performing surgery with the most modern phaco machine and implanting an IOL which is virtually free from imperfections and highly bio compatible to understand the journey made by others to come to this stage. We started cataract surgery with simple loupe, to be operated stooping, because of the focal distance of the loupe and using simple focused operation lamp for the illumination. I started using an operating microscope but that was for corneal transplants and retina surgery only. We started using operating microscope for cataract surgery much later when Extracapsular Cataract Surgery came in the fashion. Phacoemulsification came to our part of the world much later, possibly in 1991 and routine use of operating microscope also started at the same time.

While learning Cataract surgery it must be borne in mind that it is a high precision surgery and one needs to be perfect up to a millimeter to get good surgical result. Therefore repeated practice of each step is necessary until the step is mastered. It is not a difficult surgery but the surgeon has to be confident about each step before the entire surgery can be performed.

**Overview of the surgical technique**

Only five modalities will be required to be a good cataract surgeon : 1) Make up your mind 2) Get access to an Operating Microscope 3) Get access to a Phaco Machine 4) Keep an open mind, read this book, watch a lot of Videos and watch live surgeries to satisfy yourself 5) Repeat each step of the surgery many times on practice eyes until you are satisfied that you can perform the step safely.

There are lots of steps to be mastered, lots of physical maneuvers to be practiced. Every step of the surgery has to be exact; there is no scope to make mistakes. Surgery is never difficult; it is the surgeon who makes it difficult. Cataract surgery is a precision surgery and therefore, one has to master the technique. It is not enough to learn how to perform the surgery, but how perfectly and precisely one can do it.

The secret is to follow the steps exactly as strings of Pearl; each pearl has to be of the same size and type to make a perfect necklace. Time and time again we have stressed the fact that every step has a profound effect on the next step of the surgery and therefore do not proceed to the next step until the previous step has been mastered. These words cannot be repeated enough number of times to the new surgeons, but is the most important message for them.

It is very important to know the capability of the instruments and equipments well before one can start doing the surgery. There are obvious advantages of having the latest equipments, but modest equipment can do the same job if the technique is perfect. Most important advancement in the machines has become the ultrasonic power modulation and pump changes. More advancement are forthcoming in the field of cataract surgery which includes but not limited to Bimanual Micro - incision surgery, incorporation of Laser to the Phaco techniques (FEMTOSECOND LASER) and the design of the intraocular lenses to be implanted through the smallest incision possible.

One has to understand the mechanics of the steps of the surgery and practice to perform each step with precision. Cataract surgery is not only a micro surgery, it is a millimeter surgery. When each step is mastered, it is only necessary to perform each step in sequence to be a master surgeon. This book is a guide to perform the surgery and repeated practice to perform each step is required before one can be a master phaco surgeon. It is very important to learn all the techniques of cataract surgery including manual extraction of lens in addition to the phaco techniques, because a good surgeon must know when conversion is possible and necessary to avoid major complications. Therefore, I request the beginners who are keen to learn phaco surgery, should also learn SICS and ECCE surgery and learn to place and tie sutures in ocular tissue properly and understand the complications of cataract surgery in order to intervene as required during and after surgery for good surgical outcome.

**References:**

1.  WHO. int, | Priority eye diseases.
2.  *The global burden of disease : 2004 update.*. [Online-Ausg.] ed. Geneva, Switzerland: World Health *Organization; 2008. ISBN 9789241563710. p. 35.*

3. *Sperduto RD, Seigel D., Seigel D. Sperduto RD (Jul 1980). "Senile lens and senile macular changes in a population-based sample". Am J Ophthalmol 90 (1): 86–91. PMID 7395962.*

4. *Sir Harold Ridley and His Fight For Sight: He Changed the World So That We May Better See It : David J. Apple, MD SLACK Incorporated, 6900 Grove Road, Thorofare, NJ 08086.*

5. History of Phaco Surgery : Charles D. Kelman MD Phaco, Phaconit,& Laser Phaco-A quest for the best : Highlights Of Ophthalmology pp 1-8, 2002.

## Chapter 2
# THE BASIC ANATOMY OF
# THE LENS AND THE EYE

In order to perform cataract surgery, we need to have good understanding about the structure of the lens and the eye as it relates to the surgical procedure. Understanding the surgical landmarks and being aware of small distances between structures within the eye is very pertinent to cataract surgery and is important to the beginner cataract surgeon. The surgeon must understand the difference between 3 mm and 6 mm distance which may cause an excellent surgery or a disaster if this small three mm difference is not appreciated. Understanding the dimensions of all the structures for example knowing the lens is between 4 to 6 mm in thickness is very important to understand and visualize how much the phaco tip can have excursion inside this structure. Full understanding of the structures in three dimension mental image is very important for the surgeon.

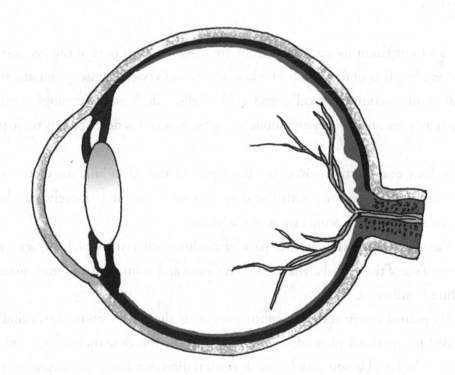

(Fig.1 Anatomy of the eye : Note the depth of the anterior chamber and the thickness of the lens and relationship of these structures to those surrounding it).

The eye is housed in the bony Orbit and is held in place by the Extraocular Muscles, Fascia and the Fat cushion which enables the eye to move smoothly within the orbit.

**The Eye Ball is made up of three coats:**

1. The Sclera and Cornea
2. The Uveal Tract composed of Choroid, Ciliary Body and the Iris
3. The Retina

The external surface of the anterior part of the globe is covered by a thin mucous membrane called the Conjunctiva. The Crystaline lens is suspended by fine Zonules which divide the eye into an anterior part and the posterior part. The Posterior part of the Eye ball is filled up with a jelly like substance, the Vitreous. The anterior part of the eye is further divided into anterior chamber and posterior chamber by the Iris. This part of the eye is filled with a liquid like substance, the Aqueous Humor. The surgeon must understand the intricate relationship of these structures and the process of healing of these structures after a surgical insult.

**The Conjunctiva:**

Conjunctiva is a transparent mucous membrane covering the front part of the eye and the inner surface of the eyelids. It contains a rich supply of fine blood vessels, dense lymphatic supply and has abundant immunocompetent cells, and goblet cells. The lymphatic supply drains to the submandibular and pre auricular lymph nodes. The conjunctiva is described in three parts:

1. **The bulbar conjunctiva** covers the front part of the sclera and the epithelium of the conjunctiva is continuous with the corneal epithelium. It is loosely attached to the underlying Tenon's Capsule except at the limbus.
2. **The Fornix conjunctiva is** that part of conjunctival layer which passes over to the undersurface of the eye lids. This part is very loose and redundant and may cause immense swelling if inflamed.
3. **The Palpebral conjunctiva** is continuous with the fornix conjunctiva and is firmly attached to the tarsal plate of the eye lid up to the mucocutaneous junction of the lid margin. The tarsal blood vessels run in vertical direction from lid margin to the fornix.

**Structure:** The conjunctiva is lined with an epithelium which is five cell layers thick and has Goblet Cells in the basal cuboidal cell layer in the infronasal area and at the fornix. This is a non keratinizing stratified squamous epithelium. Below the epithelium is a layer of loose connective tissue, the adenoid layer which is rich in blood supply from the anterior ciliary arteries, nasal artery and lachrymal artery. The substantia propria has a deep fibrous layer and is firmly attached to the tarsal plate and at the limbus, but loosely attached over the eye ball.

## Healing of wound of Conjunctiva

In experimental animals, the conjunctival injury start epithelization within 2 days in rabbits and the healing of the epithelium is complete in 3 weeks with regeneration of normal goblet cell population. Healing of the tenon's capsule is with fibroblastic hyperplasia. The conjunctiva is a friend in surgery because it can stretch considerably and can cover damaged tissues and sutures.

## Outer coat: The Sclera and Cornea:

The sclera and cornea are made up of dense fibrous tissue made up of type 1 collagen fibers. The arrangement of the collagen fibers in cornea make it optically clear. The sclera is opaque tough fibrous coat that covers posterior five sixth of the eye ball. It is thickest around the entry of the Optic Nerve and thinnest just posterior to the insertion of Extraocular Muscles.

## The Sclera:

Sclera occupies posterior five sixth of the outer coat of the eye ball. It is opaque and tough fibrous layer which gives the necessary rigidity to withstand expansion from intraocular pressure and also gives structural integrity to the eyeball. It is composed of Collagen fibers of Type I, III and V along with several types of proteoglycans in the ECM. The collagen bundles are non uniform in diameter ranging between 25 to 230 nm with run in crisscross fashion. The proteoglycan in the ECM is responsible for the hydration of the sclera which has 70% water. The sclera is opaque due to this hydration and arrangement of the Collagen fibers of which type I fibers impart structural rigidity and type V collagen gives the anchoring functions of the sclera with the adjacent structures.

Different parts of the sclera have different thickness. It is thinnest at the equator is around 0.4 mm and increases to 0.55 mm to 0.65 mm at the limbus. It is thickest at lamina cribrosa about 1.00 mm. The extraocular muscles insert with tendons which fuses with the superficial collagen of the sclera at the equator.

Episclera is a layer of dense vascular connective tissue merging with the superficial layer of the sclera which supplies most of the nutrients to this structure. It lies below the conjunctiva and tenon's capsule anteriorly and is made up of loose fibrous tissue. The Sclera proper is a tough band of collagen fibers arranged in cris - cross fashion, and not uniformly oriented. The innermost part of sclera is lamina fusca which blends with the suprachoroid lamina of the choroid.

**Development**: The sclera develops from a condensation of mesenchymal cells around the optic cup derived from neural crest cells and getting contribution from the paraxial mesoderm. The development starts at 7 weeks and continues up to 24 weeks of gestation.

**Scleral Wound Healing:**

Surgical wound healing of the sclera is important in cataract surgery. Partial thickness wound is healed within 7 to 10 days. Self sealing wound of the sclera remains open on day 1, fibroblastic tissue proliferation is seen on day 2 leading to complete healing by the 5 th day and by the 7 th day, the connective tissue is aligned with the lamellae. In my experience, scleral wound takes about 2 weeks for full healing if the wound edges are well apposed and the scleral wound is not detectable after this period. After SICS surgery, the wound margin needs to be inspected for self sealing and apposition. If the wound edges are not apposed, one stitch may be required to make it water tight and margins apposed for proper wound healing.

## THE CORNEA

The Cornea occupies the anterior one fifth of the outer coat of the eye ball. It is an avascular, transparent and tough tissue which transmits 99% of visible spectrum of light which is one of the most powerful refracting media of the eye. It is oval in shape with an average vertical diameter of 11 mm and horizontal diameter 12 mm. The radius of curvature is 7.8 mm, index of refraction 1.376 and refractive power is up to + 48 Diopters. Thickness of central cornea is 0.52 and peripheral cornea is between 0.60 to 0.65 mm. Incision for cataract surgery is confined to peripheral cornea. The surgeon has to be careful not to advance the knife to the central cornea where the thickness is less. Pachymetry to ascertain corneal thickness is an important investigation in cataract surgery. Thin or small diameter cornea pose to be a problem during the surgery and special measures may be required for the entry incision.

It is composed of five layers and recent proposed addition of Dua's layer makes it a Six layer structure with distinctive embryological origin and functional properties. The layers are: Epithelium, Bowman's Membrane, Stroma, Dua's Layer, Desmet's Membrane, and Endothelium.

**DEVELOPMENT:** As the lens vesicle detaches from the surface ectoderm at 5 to 6 weeks of gestation, this surface ectoderm gives rise to the Corneal Epithelium. A primary wave of Neural Crest Cells migrates between the Epithelium and Lens Placode at 6 weeks which gives rise to Corneal Endothelium. Mesodermal cells invading between the epithelium and endothelium is populated by a secondary wave of neural crest cells which give rise to Keratocytes that produce collagen fibers and form the corneal Stroma and other layers. Development of surface ectoderm derived corneal epithelium from 2 to 5 layers happens between 6 to 27 weeks and 7 layer thicknesses are attained at 36 weeks of gestation. The Hemidesmosomes, epithelial adhesion complexes and corneal collagen starts to develop at 9 weeks and continues up to 36 weeks. The Corneal endothelium is not a true endothelium, rather this is a neural crest derived cell layer which lines the outer side of the anterior chamber and attains the cell density, stabilizes itself by the age of 2 years after birth. The endothelial cells are not capable of cell division.

**THE EPITHELIUM:**

Corneal Epithelium is a stratified, not keratinized squamous cell layer arranged in seven layers. The basal layer of Cuboidal cells is attached to a basement membrane which is 50 to 60 nm thick and contains type IV collagen fibrils and proteoglycans. The superficial layer is shed off regularly into the tears and this turnover of the entire epithelium takes 7 days. The basal cells arise from the Limbal Stem Cells. The basal cells have hemidesmosomes which anchor them to the underlying Basement Membrane. The anchoring fibrils are made up of type VII collagen fibers which pass through the BM to the stroma. The corneal epithelium is the barrier between the Tear Film and the Stroma and allows nutrients to diffuse to the deeper layers. The epithelium along with the tear film also forms a barrier to invasion of the eye by external pathogens. As you perform refractive cataract surgery this layer becomes very important layer optically and needs meticulous evaluation regarding structural uniformity and integrity preoperatively. One has to be very careful in performing surgery in dry eye patients or in patients with sick or diseased epithelium. As we advance to perform refractive cataract surgery, careful evaluation of the epithelium is very important and is to be borne in mind.

**BOWMANS MEMBRANE:**

This is an amorphous layer beneath the Basement Membrane and is 12 microns thick. Formed of randomly arranged Collagen Fibrils of type I and is acellular. This is a modified superficial layer of the Stroma and is attached to the Epithelium by Type VII collagen fibrils which pass to the stroma.

STROMA:

The stroma makes about 90% of the corneal thickness. Structurally, it is made up of regularly arranged sheets of type I Collagen Fibrils and small amount of type V and type VI fibers. There are approximately 250 lamellas of collagen fibers which stretch to the Limbus where the fibers turn to run in circumferential direction forming an Annulus around the cornea. The curvature of the Cornea is maintained by this annulus of collagen fibrils. Elongated Keratocytes lie in between the collagen fibrils. The extracellular and extra fibrillar space is filled by proteoglycans produced by the Keratocytes. The collagen fibers are arranged in a regular fashion and interact with the proteoglycans in such a way that the whole structure do not scatter light and transmits 99% of the incident visible spectrum

Corneal stroma lies at a relatively dehydrated state and this hydration is maintained by an active transport mechanism by the endothelium. If this endothelial pump action is lost, the cornea swells due to water uptake within the stroma forms bullae under the epithelium and transparency is reduced resulting in clinical condition called corneal edema.

The transparency of the cornea is attributed to the following factors:

1. Regular arrangement of the Collagen fibrils
2. Pumping action of the Endothelium
3. Avascularity of the Cornea
4. Lateral tight junctions of the Epithelium
5. Presence of Tear Film to create a smooth surface.

**These five parameters must be maintained and assessed continually prior to and during surgery. It is important to maintain integrity of these parameters for good surgical outcomes.**

**DUA'S LAYER:**

It has been observed recently that, a very strong acellular layer of fibers is located between the Stroma and the Desmet's Membrane. This layer is 15 microns thick and is able to withstand up to 200 kPa pressure. This is believed to be part of stroma and the structure, function and significance of this layer is under investigation.

**DESMETS MEMBRANE:**

This is a thin acellular layer that is secreted by the Endothelium and serves as its basement membrane. It is composed of type IV collagen fibers and is 10 to 20 microns thick. It is firmly attached to the endothelium and may strip partly or wholly during cataract surgery along with the endothelium.

**ENDOTHELIUM:**

The corneal Endothelium is made up of a single layer of cuboidal cells which are Hexagonal in shape. The endothelial cells do not divide and if loss occurs due to disease or injury, adjacent cells expand and stretch often at the expense of their hexagonal shape to cover and compensate for the dead cells. This layer is responsible for ion and fluid transport between the stroma and the aqueous. Nutrients leak into the stroma from aqueous and water is pumped out by active transport against a concentration gradient using ATP to keep the level of hydration compatible to corneal clarity. Should breakdown happens to this barrier and the active transport system due to loss of cells by disease, toxic effect or injury, the cornea swells up and decompensate with loss of transparency.

The cell density in endothelium is between 2500 to 3000 cells/ mm3 in adults. The minimum level of cells required is 500 to 700 cells/ mm3 to maintain endothelial function.

Cataract Surgery causes loss of endothelial cells. After ICCE with A/C IOL, a 20 % cell loss occurs per year. With uncomplicated Phaco and IOL implant 8.5% cells loss occurs after one year. Higher endothelial cell loss may be due to prolonged Ultrasound time and short eye ball length. Irrigating solutions used during phaco surgery may cause cell loss if a properly buffered solution is not used. Poorly buffered solution like 0.9 % Sodium Chloride causes endothelial cell swelling and the vacuolated cells lose function which can be reversed if prolonged contact did not cause permanent damage.

Surgeon should always know the spatial relationship of the phaco tip and other instruments inside the anterior chamber and the endothelium. Any large movements or closeness of the phaco tip to the endothelium may cause permanent damage to this layer and therefore failed surgery.

## DRUG PENETRATION AND TOXICITY

Drug toxicity and penetration through cornea has strong relevance in cataract surgery.

During surgery and the post operative period the patients has to use multiple potent medications which are placed as drops on the cornea. I have experienced worst drug toxicity in my patients. Poorly buffered solutions can cause SPK and corneal ulcer and the preservatives in eye drops can cause severe allergy which is distressing both to the patients and the surgeon.

After installation of one eye drop, small amount of the medication passes through the Epithelium which allows hydrophobic lipid molecules to pass through. The Stroma allows hydrophilic molecules to pass and passage through the Endothelium is dependent on molecular size. The medication must reach the anterior chamber for its desired action to take place.

Addition of preservatives like BAK, Chlorhexidine and Thiomersal to ophthalmic preparations increases shelf life and protects the eye from infection. Most commonly used preservative is BAK (Benzalkonium Chloride). The BAK cause breakdown of bacterial cell wall, increases drug penetration, but delay wound healing. Inappropriate concentration of BAK may cause Superficial Punctate Keratopathy (SPK) and corneal ulcer. Preparation containing BAK and EDTA in appropriate concentration may safely be used in normal patients. In patients with diseased cornea, preservative free eye drops limits the potential damage that it may cause to the epithelium.

All preservatives may cause damage to corneal endothelium and should never be introduced into the A/C. Preservative free Xylocaine, Epinephrine 1:1000 and Pilocarpine have been used in the Anterior chamber during surgery. The effect of these preservative free drugs on the corneal endothelium is reversible.

If drug allergy is suspected with any topical ophthalmic medication, the product should be stopped immediately and replaced by preservative free alternate medications.

## HEALING OF CORNEAL WOUND

Healing of corneal epithelium depends upon the type of injury. When the epithelium is injured by abrasion or removed surgically, the adjacent cells enlarge and migrate laterally to cover the defect and then cell division in the basal layer starts to bring back the stratified squamous structure. Epithelial wound of 6 mm diameter heals within 48 hours. After wound healing, new hemidesmosomes are formed to ensure adhesion of the basal layer to the Basement membrane. When abrasion occurs sparing the basement membrane, hemidesmosomes appear and normal architecture is quickly reestablished. When injury involves removal of the basement membrane, the basal layers must secret a new basement membrane and then create new hemidesmosomes which may take 12 to 18 months. This is important to remember the healing period during the treatment of Corneal Erosion and iatrogenic removal of epithelium during surgery.

Wound healing of the Stroma is different. Following penetrating injury to the stroma, the wound is immediately populated by leucocytes. The keratocytes undergo modification and proliferation to produce collagen fibrils and proteoglycans which are laid down to create a scar. The healed corneal stromal wound is not optically clear because the newly produced fibers may not be regularly arranged. The resulting scar may take up to 4 years or longer to build up tensile strength.

Desmet's Membrane when detached from the stroma heals up quickly if the detachment is small. In large detachment it takes longer to heal and may result in decompensation of the endothelium with resulting corneal edema.

The Cells of Endothelium layer are incapable of cell division. Therefore, if there is injury to endothelium resulting in loss of cells, the defect is covered quickly by elongation and migration of cells from adjacent area and the pump function is returned. The pump action and barrier function are re-established once the wounded area is healed and continuous single layer of endothelial cells are established. When the loss of cell is so much that, the number of endothelial cells falls short of the critical count, the cornea becomes edematous and decompensate and therefore needs replacement by a corneal graft. This fact is to be remembered during Phaco surgery and the surgeon has to limit the endothelial cell loss due to Ultrasound use by coating it with good quality viscoelastics and other measures which will be discussed in subsequent chapters. Use of appropriate irrigating solutions is also another important thing to remember during phaco surgery because improper solutions can damage the endothelial cells.

## SURGICAL LANDMARKS:

**Limbus:** This is the transition zone between the Cornea in and Sclera. The bulbar conjunctiva is firmly attached to the underlying structures at the limbus. The clear corneal lamellae become continuous with circular and oblique opaque fibbers of the Sclera. The surgical Limbus is a 2 mm wide zone with clear cornea on one side and opaque sclera on the other side. Limbus is an important landmark for entry to the anterior chamber. Form anterior to posterior they are:

A. The Blue Limbal Zone: This is the bluish translucent transitional zone of the periphery of the cornea just behind the anterior limbal border. This is about 1 mm in width.

B. Mid- Limbal Zone: This is the junction between the blue zone with the white sclera. It overlies termination of Desmet's membrane (Schwalbe's Line) on the inside.

C. Posterior Limbal Border: This lies 1 mm posterior to the mid- limbal line and overlies scleral spur on the inside.

D. White Limbal Zone: This is 1 mm wide zone in the Opaque sclera behind the posterior limbal border and overlies the Trabecular Meshwork.

## CATARACT INCISIONS:

Several types are cataract incisions are practiced they are:

1. Scleral incision: This is located behind the posterior limbal border and attached conjunctiva is to be dissected to gain access to the sclera. Bleeding may occur while conjunctival incision is given and scleral dissection performed.

2. Posterior Limbal Incision: This is located at the white limbal zone between the mid limbal line and the posterior limbal border. The underlying Trabecular meshwork may be injured

3. Mid-Limbal Incision : This incision is given at the mid-limbal line which corresponds to the Schwalbe's line internally

4. Anterior Limbal Incision: This incision is located in the Blue limbal zone and traverses the Desmet's membrane. It may cause stripping of Desmet's membrane and therefore caution is to be applied.

5. Clear Corneal Incision: This is located in front of the blue line anterior to the limbus. This may also be associated with stripping of the Desmet's membrane.

6. Limbal Incision during ECCE surgery is at the surgical limbus.

## THE ANTERIOR CHAMBER

The anterior chamber is a small space between the endothelium of the cornea in front and Iris behind. It measures 2.06 to 3.62 mm as measured by ultrasound A scan and IOL Master biometry. In Emmetropes the depth is approximately 3.16 to 3.56 mm, in Hypermetropes it is shallower 2.5 to 2.7 mm and in Myopes it measures 3.16 to 3.56. In children, the depth is shallower. It is important to realize the fact that, during Phaco Surgery or any form of Cataract Surgery, the surgeon has to work within this limited space for instrumentation and Irrigation and Aspiration. **Excursion of the phaco tip within this small space requires very steady hand and collapse of the anterior chamber can cause damage to the structures above it or below it.**

The anterior chamber is filled with Aqueous Humor which is formed by ultrafiltration and active transport at the Ciliary Body. It enters the posterior chamber, flows around the lens, passes through the pupil to the anterior chamber and leaves the eye through the Trabecular Meshwork at the angle of the anterior chamber. Very little fluid also passes by Uveoscleral Outflow. The rate of formation and drainage of Aqueous is approximately 2.5 micro liters / minute.

Composition of the aqueous humor is important in phacosurgery. In pre phaco days, during the 1970s, we rarely needed to use irrigating solutions in the anterior chamber except for unlikely complication of breaking the anterior capsule during ICCE resulting in unplanned EECE, or during Needling and aspiration of congenital cataracts. BSS was not available and Sodium Chloride Saline when used for irrigation cause swelling of the Endothelium, and therefore, we were careful not to use this for prolonged period and cause permanent damage to the endothelium.

During modern age phaco surgery, irrigating solution needs to be circulating in the anterior chamber during emulsification of the nucleus or irrigation and aspiration of the cortical mater. This requires the use of irrigating solutions that is close to aqueous in composition. The aqueous is close to plasma in composition with the difference that, it has less protein and high concentration of Ascorbic acid which is 20 times higher and high concentration of lactate. Other substances which are present in Aqueous are, Glutathione, Calcium and Bicarbonate. Thus, the solution which has the closest composition to aqueous is BSS PLUS. The other solution which is compatible to endothelial health is Ringer Lactate with Glutathione and Bicarbonate (GBR) solution.

The solution should have a pH between 6.7 and 8.1 and Osmolarity between 270 to 350 m osml/L.

## THE UVEAL TRACT

Anatomy of the uveal tract is important for the cataract surgeon not only because it is the most important coat supplying nutrients to the structures of the eye but also because of the fact that part of this layer, the iris plays an important role during cataract surgery.

The uveal tract is a vascular layer between the outer sclera and the inner coat, the retina. It is heavily pigmented layer that blocks light rays to pass through and act as the black interior coating of the camera allowing sharp image of the objects to fall on the retina.

It has three parts, from the front to back they are, Iris, Ciliary Body and the Choroid. However, the whole uveal tract developmentally, structurally and functionally acts as a single unit.

### Development:

The uveal tract develops partly from the neuroectoderm layer of the optic cup and partly from the condensation of the mesoderm around the Optic cup.

At 9 weeks of gestation the ciliary body starts to develop.

At 12 weeks, the Sphincter pupillae muscles of the iris develop from the neuroectoderm.

At 5 months of gestation, all layers of the uveal tract are visible.

At 6 months, the Dilator pupillae muscle starts to develop while Sphincter Pupillae is fully developed.

Development of all the layers and muscles including the pigment cells are completed and attains adult proportion by the age of 5 years.

Both layers of ciliary and iris epithelium develops from the two layers of the optic cup while the stroma of the iris and ciliary body and choroid develops form the Mesodermal condensation around the optic cup.

## IRIS

The Iris is a diaphragm, a shallow cone cut at the apex to form the pupil. It hangs from the anterior part of the ciliary body between the cornea and the lens dividing the anterior part of the eye into anterior chamber and posterior chamber and immersed in aqueous humor. It has an average diameter of 12 mm and thickness of 0.5 mm. The pupillary aperture is 3 to 4 mm in diameter and is dependent on the parasympathetic and sympathetic tone. The iris is thinnest at the root and very easily tears off from ciliary body giving rise to Iridodialysis.

The iris has a stroma which lies anteriorly and contains the blood vessels, nerves and the sphincter and dilator pupillae muscle along with loose areolar tissue and pigment cells.

Behind the stroma there are two layers of epithelium. Anterior epithelium is derived from the outer layer of the optic cup and is attached to the dilator pupillae muscle. The posterior epithelial layer is derived from the inner layer of the optic cup and curves up through the pupil for a short distance to form the pigment frill on the surface of the iris. Sphincter pupillae is supplied by the parasympathetic nerves through the ciliary ganglion and contraction causes constriction of the pupil. The dilator pupillae is supplied by the Sympathetic nerves of the internal carotid sympathetic plexus and causes dilatation of the pupil. The pharmacological properties of the pupil are important because, the phaco surgery must be performed through a dilated pupil.

The stroma of the iris contains blood vessels which form two arterial circles. The two long ciliary arteries proceed forward through the ciliary body and together with branches from the anterior ciliary arteries form the Major Arterial circle. Branches from this arterial circle and the anterior ciliary arteries form another minor arterial circle at the iris border.

The iris is a very vascular structure and surgical injury to the stroma may cause severe bleeding leading to hyphaema. Accidental suction of the iris by the phaco tip may cause tear and total disinsertion of the iris. Surgical cut injury to the iris can be repaired by sutures but the injury is not healed by any process of repair or regeneration.

## THE CILIARY BODY

The ciliary body is directly continuous with the Iris in front and Choroid behind. The ciliary body serves three important functions. They are 1) Suspension of the Lens by zonular fibers, 2)

Accommodation of the eye by changing the radius of curvature of the lens by contraction of the ciliary muscles. 3) Secretion of aqueous humor.

The ciliary body extends from the scleral spur to about 7.5 mm behind the limbus on the temporal side and 6.5 mm on the nasal side. It has two parts, 1) Pars Plicata which is anterior 2.5 mm and has 70 to 80 ciliary processes, and 2) Pars Plana posterior 3mm which is smooth and is a continuation of the layers of the choroids.

Structurally, the ciliary body consists of stroma and epithelium. The stroma is composed of loosely arranged collagen fibers which aggregate around the muscles and ciliary processes. Ciliary muscles are arranged in bundles of Longitudinal fibers, Circular fibers and Radial fibers, supplied by the parasympathetic fibers from ciliary ganglion. Rest of the stroma contains blood vessels which constitute the Major Arterial Circle and its tributaries.

The epithelium has two layers; a) Pigmented Epithelium is the anterior of the two epithelial layers and is continuous with RPE. b) Non pigmented epithelial layer which is posterior of the two layers and gives attachment to the Zonular Fibers.

The ciliary processes are 70 to 80 in number each about 2 mm long. Each has a central core of capillaries surrounded by a stroma and the two layers of the ciliary epithelium. Tight junction between the epithelial cells constitutes the blood aqueous barrier. A basement membrane lies between the two epithelium layers.

## THE CHOROID:

The choroid is a thin vascular pigmented lamina that occupies posterior five – sixth of the middle layer of the coats of the eye ball. It is firmly attached to the sclera with supra choroids lamina, Lamina Fusca and internally attached to the Retinal Pigment Epithelium (RPE). It is thin anteriorly being only 0.1 mm and thicker posteriorly about 0.22 mm

The chorid is described in three layers, 1) Outer layer of small blood vessels with loose connective tissue, 2) Layer of Chorio Capillaries 3) Bruch's membrane

The vascular supply is from short posterior ciliary arteries. The two Long Posterior ciliary arteries pass forward to the ciliary body to form the Major Arterial Circle of the Iris.

The venous drainage is through the four Vortex veins that pierce the choroids and sclera 6 mm behind the equator. The two superior vortex veins drain in the superior ophthalmic vein, the two inferior vortex veins drain into the inferior ophthalmic vein.

The function of the uveal tract is to supply blood and nutrients to the outer layer of the eye ball. This layer has immunocompetent cells and inflammation cause outpouring of the inflammatory cells and protein in to the anterior chamber and vitreous giving rise to Iritis, Cyclitis, or Pan uveitis.

## THE LENS

The lens is the structure on which Phaco Surgery is performed. Therefore, full knowledge of the structure and function of the lens is very important to a cataract surgeon. Crystalline lens is a transparent biconvex structure surrounded by a capsule and is suspended behind the iris from the Ciliary Body by zonular fibers. Together with the Cornea it aids in refraction of light so that sharp images are formed on the retina. The lens is capable of changing its power by a mechanism called, accommodation.

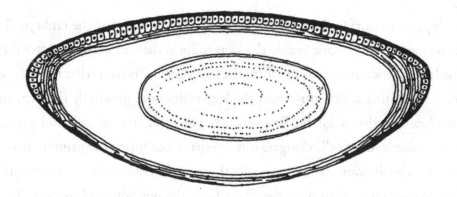

(Fig 2. The lens. Note the structure of the Lens and Epithelium, Cortex Nucleus and the capsules of the lens).

Horizontal diameter of lens is: 9 to 10 mm. Antero posterior thickness is 4.5 to 6 mm and Diopteric power: +18 to +22 D.

**It is important to know and understand the thickness of the lens which is 4 to 6 mm and therefore the small amount of movement the phaco tip is capable to perform within this**

distance in order to remove the lens. It is worthwhile to measure on a caliper 4 mm and 6 mm and physically realize how much the distance is where the phaco tip can safely be manipulated.

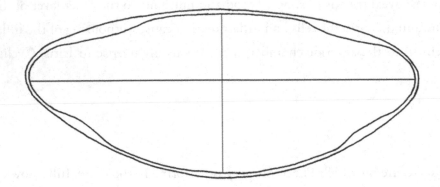

**(Fig 3 the thickness of the lens: Note the thickness or anterio-posterior diameter of the lens which is 4-5 mm. The surgeon can move the phaco tip through this distance.)**

**Development:**

The lens develops from Surface Ectoderm that lines the head part of the embryo. The surface ectoderm at the mouth of the optic vesicle thickens to form the lens Placode. After the optic cup is formed, the lens Placode transforms to form the lens vesicle. The cells that form the lens vesicle secret a thin basal lamina which surrounds the lens vesicle and gradually thickens to form the Capsule of the Lens. At this stage, the lens vesicle has anterior layer of cells and a posterior layer of cells. The posterior layer of cells elongate fills the space and forms the primary lens fibers. The anterior epithelium proliferates rapidly specially those at the equator elongates, acquires protein Crystaline and passes forward to meet the fibers from the opposite end to form the secondary lens fibers which ultimately forms the lens cortex and the nucleus while the primary fibers are gradually replaced.

**FORMATION OF LENS FIBERS**

The lens fibers constitute the bulk portion of the lens and its differentiation and formation is a complex process. The first step in the differentiation is withdrawal from the cell cycle. The cells migrate from the germinative zone to the transitional zone, acquire crystalline and degrade the nucleus along with all membrane bound organelles and specialization of the plasma membrane leads to elongation and formation the lens fibers.

The fibers elongate, meet the fibers of the opposite side at the Y sutures. Inside the fibers this contains high amount of protein Crystalline, Glutathione and Ascorbic acid. Individual lens fibers are 4-7 micron in diameter and up to 12 mm long. The lens fibers at the center of the lens are compressed. Successive layers of lens fibers are laid down throughout life.

## FORMATION OF THE CAPSULE:

In early embryonic life when the lens vesicle is formed, the cells lay down a basement membrane. During invagination, this basal lamina comes to surround the lens vesicle which thickens, acquires type IV collagen fibers and proteoglycans to form the lens capsule in the adult lens

## STRUCTURE OF THE LENS:

The lens has four arbitrary parts, 1) Capsule, 2) Lens Cortex, 3) Epinucleus, 4) Nucleus

## THE CAPSULE:

The capsule of the lens is homogenous and transparent structure which closely surrounds the lens. The anterior part of the capsule is thicker about 12 to 14 microns that the posterior part about 3.5 to 4 microns. It is thickest at the equator 21 microns where the Zonular fibers are inserted. It is highly elastic and is composed of type IV collagen fibers. A single layer of cells line the inner surface to the anterior capsule which contributes to the formation of the lens fibers. When ruptured or torn, the edges roll up and curl away which cannot be repaired or regenerate. It is important to note that, the lens capsule is non forgiving and if torn, results in failed surgery.

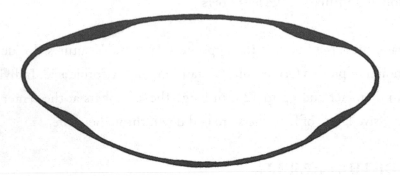

(Fig 4. The lens Capsule: Note the thickness of the capsule which is 4
Micron at the posterior pole and 14 Microns at the anterior capsule)

## THE ZONULES:

The zonules are special structures which keep the lens suspended from the ciliary body. They are attached to the capsule of the lens near the equator and continuous with the basal lamina of the non pigmented epithelial layer of the ciliary body. The attachment of the zonular fibers extends 2 to 2.5 mm on the anterior capsule and 1.5 mm in the posterior capsule. Thus on the flat surface of the anterior capsule, about 6 to 6.5 mm area is available for safe capsulorhexis. If the Rhexis extends beyond 6 mm, it has a tendency to proceed along the zonular fibers to the posterior capsule. The zonular fibers are made up of Fibrillin and are strong in young age getting weaker with advancing age and stress on the zonules may cause rupture and prolapse of the entire lens into the anterior chamber, the property which had been utilized in the past to perform Intracapsular Cataract Extraction (ICCE) with Cryo machine. Use of new prostate medications we can get weak zonules and the surgeon has to be on the guard while operating on these patients because of zonular weakness.

## CORTEX:

The cortex is formed of recently developed lens fibers that sweep behind the capsule to meet the fibers of the opposite side at the anterior and posterior Y sutures. The cortex is soft and can be aspirated easily with a cannula or the I/A tip of the phaco machine. The bulk of the cortex is determined by the age of the lens.

## EPI NUCLEUS:

The epi nucleus is the deposition of lens fibers surrounding the central nucleus and can be cut easily and can be removed by aspiration by I/A probe or the phaco probe by aspiration only. It requires more aspiration power to remove than the cortex. If a wave of BSS is passed between the nucleus and epi- nucleus, they can be separated and demarcated by the fluid wave.

## NUCLEUS:

The nucleus is formed of compressed lens fibers. As lens fibers are laid down, old fibers are compressed in the center of the lens which progressively becomes harder. In early life, the nucleus is soft in consistency but as age progress, this becomes progressively harder and after formation of cataract, this cannot be removed by aspiration. It requires fragmentation and emulsification for removal through a small incision. During surgery as you phaco deeper, one can see through the microscope the alteration in the texture of the lens which changes from a rough texture of the nucleus to a smooth texture of the cortex. This means that, the groove is deep enough.

## TRANSPARENCY OF THE LENS:

It is important that the lens remains clear for the required refraction and vision. This is accomplished due to the presence of protein Crystalline and the absence of cellular organelles in the lens fibers. The lens is a partially dehydrated structure with water content of about 66 % and this dehydrated status is accomplished by active transport of ions across the lens capsule.

## NUTRITION:

The lens gets its nutrition from the aqueous humor. Glucose metabolism occurs in the anaerobic pathway in the fibers and aerobic respiration occurs in the epithelial cells. The other nutrients move across the lens capsule from the aqueous by diffusion and active transport.

## FORMATION OF CATARACT:

### Nuclear Cataract:

Age related changes are the most important factors in the production of nuclear cataract. It accounts for 60% of all age related cataracts. The nucleus of the lens may assume greenish white or brunescent tinge which cause light scattering. Oxidative damage of the lens proteins, altered Glutathione metabolism and loss of ascorbate may be accountable for the changes that lead to the formation of the opacities. When left untreated, the nuclear cataracts become harder and change color from greenish to yellowish to amber color and finally become black or brown in color and very large and hard in consistency or turn into white milky liquid with a hard nucleus.

**Cortical Cataract:**

In cortical cataract formation, the mature lens fibers close to the surface are affected. Initially, the damage to a small number of fibers at a localized area of the cortex is evident. This damage is multifactorial and results is the disruption of ion pumps, accumulation of intracellular Ca+ causing damage to cell membranes and coagulation of the protein results in the formation of the opacities. Extension of the opacity over the total length of an area of fiber cells causes the clinical shape of Cortical Spokes. The cortical opacities may also spread around the lens circumference. The cellular damage and disruption of the protein gives rise to a Chalky White appearance of these opacities. Localized trauma to the lens fibers either mechanical or chemical also leads to the formation of cortical cataracts.

**Posterior Sub-Capsular Cataracts (PSC):**

This is a special form of cataract develops due to certain reasons like Steroid use, Chemotherapy and Diabetes mellitus. A collection of swollen cells at the center of the posterior pole just beneath the capsule develop and these opaque cells scatter light. Since these opacities lie at the optical axis, these opacities cause early deterioration of vision. This may be associated with cortical or nuclear cataract. Whatever may be the cause or type, they require early surgery to restore clear optical axis for vision.

## VITREOUS

Vitreous is a transparent jelly like substance that occupies the posterior part of the eyeball. It forms a semisolid support for the retina and mechanically stabilizes it. Total volume of the vitreous is about 4 ml and the water content is 98 % to 99.7 % is a hydrogel with a refractive index of 1.3348 and allows 90% of visible light to pass.

**Development:**

During development, three stages are evident. 1) The primary vitreous,

2) The secondary vitreous 3) The tertiary vitreous or zonules.

In the fifth week of development, the space between the lens and the optic vesicle is filled with vascularized mesoderm. During sixth week, the hyaloid artery is developed and nourishes the lens vesicle. Secondary vitreous starts to develop by the ninth week. By the seventh month the primary vitreous atrophies and the secondary vitreous fills the cavity. By the time of birth, the hyaloid artery is reabsorbed leaving behind Cloquet's canal. The tertiary vitreous or the zonules begins to form in the 6 the month partially from the vitreous and partly from the basement membrane of the ciliary epithelium.

## Structure of the vitreous:

Vitreous is composed of a network of randomly arranged collagen fibrils and hyaluronic acids forming a hydrogel in which some cells called, the vitreocytes are present. The vitreous has a cortical zone and a central core vitreous. The collagen network is prominent in the Cortex and less pronounced in the core vitreous. The cortical vitreous is firmly attached to the periphery of the retina at ora serrata and around the optic disc. It is also attached around the macula and blood vessels. The core vitreous may undergo liquefaction and degeneration due to age, disease or trauma. The vitreous base may get detached from the retina causing PVD. Hemorrhage or opacities in the vitreous may need removal by vitrectomy. Vitrectomy may also be necessary to treat retinal detachment.

## Surgical Importance:

1) If the posterior capsule of the lens is broken during cataract surgery, the vitreous prolepses through the broken capsule into the anterior chamber. The vitreous is a gel like substance and because of the presence of the collagen fibrils, it acts like a Slinky. The more it is pulled; more vitreous comes out causing collapse of the globe. Therefore, the protruding vitreous must be cut by closed vitrectomy. This fact must be remembered during cataract surgery. Sponge vitrectomy should never be done and no pull should be exerted on the vitreous strands which are in the anterior chamber. The surgery should be stopped immediately and closed chamber anterior vitrectomy or pars plana vitrectomy should be performed by a vitrector or vitrectomy machine.

2) When cataract surgery is performed on an eye which has undergone vitrectomy surgery before, it is necessary to remember that, the replaced vitreous is not a gel and therefore, cannot give the necessary firm support to the lens during surgery.

The eye must be filled with good viscoelastic for capsulorhexis and a forceps rhexis is better. Also the whole surgery needs to be performed with low flow, low power mode which necessitates modification of the machine parameters.

## THE RETINA

The retina is the light-sensitive layer composed of neural cells and is the innermost of the three coats of the eyeball. It is attached to the Choroid externally and lined internally by the Vitreous body which is firmly attached to the retina at certain areas. The optics of the eye (Cornea and Lens) creates images on the retina specially the Macula and fovea necessary for vision. Light striking the retina initiates a series of chemical and electrical events that ultimately trigger nerve impulses which are transmitted to the brain through the Optic Nerve to produce visual sensation.

The retina and the optic nerve originate as outgrowths of the developing neural tube and the two layers of the Optic Cup.

The retina has ten distinct layers of cells interconnected by synapses. The only neurons that are directly sensitive to light are the Rods and Cones. Rods function mainly in dim light and provide black-and-white vision, while cones support daytime vision and the perception of color.

Neural signals from the rods and cones undergo processing by other neurons of the retina. The output takes the form of action potentials in retinal ganglion cells whose axons form the optic nerve and these signals are transmitted to the brain.

## RETINA IN CATARACT SURGERY:

Retina suffers various insults during cataract surgery some of which are reversible, some are not. It is important for the surgeon to understand these situations and detect and manage the conditions as they occur.

**During Surgery:** 1) Injury to the photoreceptors by the Microscope light has been documented. The microscope light is a condensed light and falls on the macula during surgery. Therefore, the light intensity is to be modified during the course of surgery to minimize this effect. While the cataractous lens is present, little light can pass through and higher intensity is not likely to cause any damage. However, as the lens is emulsified, microscope light hits the macula with full intensity. The light intensity is to be reduced or blocked when the surgeon is not working on the eye.

2) In the event of break of the posterior capsule, the vitreous prolapse through the broken capsule. If traction is applied on the vitreous, the retina may break and cause retinal detachment.

**Post Operatively:** 1) Vitreous degeneration and liquefaction may cause traction on the macula and cause cystoid macular edema (CME) in the postoperative period. 2) Diabetic Maculopathy may cause poor vision in the postoperative period after successful phaco surgery and IOL implantation.

**REFERENCES:**

1. Conjunctival epithelial wound healing : Harry S Geggel, Judith Friend and Richard A. Thaft : Invest Ophthalmol Vis Sci 25: 860-863, 1984

2. Thoft R A and Friend J : The XYZ hypothesis of corneal epithelial maintance, Invest Ophthalmol Vis Sci 24: 1442, 1983

3. Hanna CX and O Brian JE : Cell Production and Migration in the epithelial layer of cornea : Arch Ophthalmology : 64-563, 1960

4. HS Dua, JAP Gomes, A Singh : Corneal Epithelial Wound healing, British Journal of Ophthalmology, 1994; 78: 401-408

5. Adler's Physiology of the Eye Clinical Application : Tenth Edition, Edited by Paul L. Kaufman and Albert Alm ; Mosby 200324

6. Rafael I. Barraquer, Ralph Michael, Rodrigo Abreu, Jose Lamarca and Francisco Tresserra :

   Human Lens Capsule Thickness as a Function of Age and Location along the Sagittal Lens Peremeter 10.1167/iovs.05-1002 Invest. Ophthalmol. Vis. Sci. May 2006 vol.47 no 5 2053-2060

# Chapter 3
# THE MICROSCOPE AND INSTRUMENTS

Operating Microscope is one of the most essential equipments necessary for Eye Surgery. When I started Eye Surgery back in 1973, we could operate using the Ophthalmic Loupe and work standing. The surgery used to be Cryo Extraction of the Lens in Intracapsular Cataract Operation with 8/0 Virgin Silk sutures. We would need to use the microscope rarely, but very quickly, during the end of the decade, Intraocular Lens Implantation was started and using a Microscope was necessary.

Now it is mandatory to learn and get accustomed with an Operating Microscope and also important to learn Eye –Hand coordination, Eye-Hand-Foot coordination and learn to use the non dominant hand and foot.

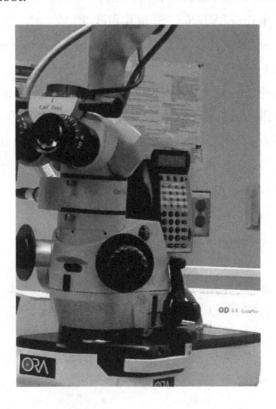

(Fig. 5. The Microscope : Note that the Knobs are all covered by sterile covers and needs to be changed for each surgery)

There are many makes and models of the Operating Microscope, some less expensive and some are highly expensive. All claiming to be the best and this may be overwhelming for the beginner surgeon. Any operating microscope which has good Illumination, manual or automatic zoom, foot focusing control, has coaxial illumination and good depth of focus, is adequate for Cataract surgery. I found it quiet easy to adapt to the Surgical Microscope. All that will be required is patience, practice and learn a few maneuvers to perform microsurgery. While looking through the microscope, the surgeon is stationary, the instruments and equipments have to be handled in a few specific manners with controlled and deliberate movements. This part of the learning process is difficult and until the maneuvers of how to use the instruments under the microscope with continuous focusing control is mastered, no eye surgery should be contemplated. To an eye surgeon it is not a big deal to use the microscope, but I know and can feel how much difficult it may be for the beginner to adapt to a complex equipment like an Operating Microscope.

There are many companies that manufacture the operating microscopes. The optics also varies a lot from one company to the other. Basically there are four parts of the equipment:

1. The Eye Piece
2. The Magnification
3. Focusing control
4. Illumination control.

Some microscopes have eye piece setting so that there is a distance between eye piece and the eye; others need to be adjusted so that the eye is very near to the eye-piece. Check it while adjusting the eye piece. The eye piece also has surgeon's refractive correction. Set it at '0" for the start. The Interpupillary distance (IPD) is the next important setting.

Close one eye & look at the field and then the other, to confirm that the object in focus is equally sharp with each eye. If not, adjust the eye pieces by rotating the eye piece to change the refractive correction. When the object is equally clear with either eye, set the Interpupillary distance (IPD) with both eyes open and adjust the IPD setting. Different microscopes have different tools for adjusting the IPD. The object now should be clearly visible with both eyes open and with depth perception this means that you must be able to see the top and bottom part of the objet in view at the same time. Some surgeons may have a Phoria and Exophoria is more common. This has to be compensated by adjusting the IPD. Fusion of the images with two eyes open is essential. Practice this for a couple of days with the microscope you intend to use. If it is not possible to get fusion and steriopsis by adjusting the eye piece, talk to an Ophthalmologist, you may need a small Prism correction and use glasses to compensate for your phoria.

**Seating:**

The surgeon must be seated comfortably on an adjustable stool; the Operating Table must also be adjustable and suited to surgeons comfort.

Never sit at a position where you have to stretch your neck to look through the eye piece of the microscope, sit comfortably as if sitting on your favorite stool at home. Next adjust the stool height so that your feet can comfortably reach the microscope focusing control with the left foot and the Foot Paddle of the Phaco machine on the floor with your Right Foot. If your feet are not touching the floor comfortably, lower the stool and the operating Table to your height, sit erect and look through the eye piece, some microscopes have movable eye piece control so that it can be adjusted to your eye height, some do not have this adjustment. You should be able to look at the cornea, the anterior chamber and the red reflex at your comfortable posture. I once worked at hospital where all the other surgeons were at least 7 inch taller than me. Believe me, it used to be extremely difficult for me to adjust the microscope at that operation room and I had hard time to operate at that center. Learn this adjustment before you start to learn eye surgery.

To start with, begin at the lowest magnification. I find 5 x magnifications for basic surgeries satisfactory. If you need higher magnifications, you can now change to higher magnification and use the focusing control to focus at every step. The microscope may have a foot control for focusing. It should be at the appropriate place. It is important to start at medium illumination at the beginning & then adapt to brighter and higher or lower illumination. The surgeon must be seated comfortably on an adjustable tool with the operation table adjusted to the comfort of the surgeon, sit erect & look down the microscope. To minimize tremor of the hands, forearms & hands need to be supported. The operation table should be designed for this comfort. Tremor varies with individuals and operating conditions. I never get a tremor while operating. But if I become conscious regarding the importance of my patient say, some of my relatives, I get a tremor & shakiness. It is true that surgical results are always good if the surgeon is relaxed.

While adapting to the microscope, try to perform minor operations or tying sutures under microscope first.

Next, before performing cataract surgery, you need to adapt to higher magnification and greater depth of focus. So the beginner surgeon must learn to adjust the zoom control and focusing control. Take the microscope to higher zoom and bring the microscope down until the edge of Iris is visible. Now adjust the Zoom Control and focusing control to properly to gain maximum clarity and depth of focus. It is a common mistake to use zoom of the microscope while structures are not in focus. The simple point is, if the structure is not in sharp focus in high magnification, you cannot perform surgery on that structure.

I should not be suggesting how a particular surgeon will get used to the microscope, but I was advised by my mentor at the beginning of Microsurgery when microscopes were rarely used, to shave with the right hand for a week and then shave with the left hand for a week. Try to write alphabets with the left non dominant hand and look at instruments through the microscope while holding instruments with the left hand. Then he suggested me to peel potatoes with potato peeler under the microscope. This was because; using instruments under the microscope by an inexperienced hand may cause injury to the eye. Dr. Mehdi Vazeen MD suggested practicing different steps of the surgery on Grapes. Grapes give a firm surface to practice Capsulorhexis and also phaco chop. One can also practice tying sutures on grapes. I prefer to use goats or pigs eyes for practice. Cadaver eyes are better alternative but hard to get. During my learning phase, practiced a lot on Goats eyes mounted on a holder devised by me and held stationary by the nurse. I learned incision, Capsulorhexis, hydrodissection, groove and chip and flip technique on goat's eyes. I also practiced tying sutures under the microscope using goat's eyes.

Now you are comfortably seated, with the microscope adjusted to the minimum magnification, focused correctly, and the surgical field is within your vision. Look through the eye piece to be sure that you can see everything. Next take a scissors and a forceps at your hands & bring it into the microscopic field and look through the eye-piece again you will see the instruments clearly. Gradually lower the instrument down to the surgical object like conjunctiva catch it with forceps in the left hand, cut it with scissors in the right hand & when this is complete, go out of the microscopic field and hand over the instruments to the nurse.

Take the next instrument & follow the same procedure throughout the surgery. During this learning curve, you will alternately see outside the microscopic field with bare eyes and through the microscope at the microscopic field. Over a period of time, with practice, you will easily learn to perform the whole surgery looking through the microscope. Just put your hand forward for the instrument you require & once it is placed between your fingers; gently bring it to the operating field. Be slow and deliberate in your movements. Don't panic, don't rush, & have patience. If you make a small injury to the corneal epithelium, while stitching for example, it will look horrifying under the microscope. Don't worry, this will heal up. Your movements should be slow so that even if you make a tissue injury with the instrument, the injury is minimum and cause no harm to the patient. The instruments should be an extension of your fingers and you should be able to feel the instrument's resistance on the tissue.

Try to perform the surgery you know the best for example, pterygium excision or Chalazion Incision under the microscope. Once you are confident, you can perform all surgeries under the microscope, do some practice with Goats eyes or Cadaver eyes from the Eye bank, before you start cataract surgery.

Once you have practiced with superficial surgeries you will be confident to make a move towards performing intraocular surgery like ECCE or SICS or Phaco Surgery.

One important thing is control of the hand to handle sharp instruments, please don't use sharp blades or diamond knife until you are fully confident that you have control over the movement of your hands and they are fully supported.

It is important to practice daily to be proficient with the microscope. Your next move should be to practice tying sutures. Cataract surgery is largely no suture surgery in the present time. But you will need to learn suturing because, you may have to convert to ECCE or may need to insert one or two sutures if there is a wound leak. This requires some practice.

## Tying Sutures

You have to practice tying sutures under the microscope. This requires specific micro instruments and specific maneuvers.

While tying sutures, you will find that, because of diminished field, you cannot see one end of the suture while you bring the other end in view. You have to make the loops within the field of your vision and therefore, you cannot hold the suture anywhere between your fingers and make the loop as you can do without the microscope.

Always tie sutures at low magnification in the beginning. While placing sutures, hold the needle correctly with your micro needle holder outside the microscopic field.

Then bring the toothed forceps to hold the tissue within your microscopic field. Hold the tissue & pass the needle at the correct plane & bring it out. Now pull the suture out & keep pulling while looking through the microscope until you can see the other free end of the suture. Pull gently or other end of the suture will go out of the wound before you know it. Leave the suture there.

Now you hold the needle again with the needle holder in the correct orientation and bring the needle in the operating field pass the needle through the other tissue you want to tie with the first one. Next pull the suture which should be passing smoothly through both the tissues until the other end of the suture is visible under the microscope and the two tissue ends are apposed. Now take a micro-tying forceps in your left hand and another micro tying forceps in your right hand. You can use toothed forceps with tying platform if you like. Next hold the long end of the stitch within the microscopic field with the forceps in your left hand. Using the forceps in your right hand, make two loops over this end of the suture. Now pick up the other free end of the suture with the tying forceps in your right hand within the microscopic field & gently tie. It is easy to do this but requires some practice.

While using 8/0 suture you should take two turns for the first loop, one turn for the second loop. This will tie the suture satisfactorily. Be careful not to tighten the suture too tight. The tension should be adequate for keeping the wound edges in apposition. If sutures are too loose or too tight, they should be removed & re - sutured.

It is more difficult to handle 10/0 Nylon sutures. 10/0 Nylon suture gives rise to less tissue reaction and epithelium can grow over the nylon and this can be left alone buried inside the tissue. However, it is wiser to delay its use until suturing with 8/0 has been completely mastered. You may next try 9/0 Nylon before mastering 10/0 Monofilament Nylon. While tying the 10/0 Nylon interrupted suture, follow the same procedure as tying with 8/0 virgin silk. The only difference is in tying the knot and cutting the ends.

Because 10/0 Nylon knot tends to slip, the first loop should be tied with three turns, second with two turns and a third with one turn. This will give a very satisfactory knot. The loops need to be tightened adequately otherwise the stitch will loosen & cause the knot to give away.

The next important thing is to cut the suture end. The exposed 10/0 nylon suture end if kept long may pierce the conjunctival epithelium & then act like a knife to irritate the conjunctiva at the undersurface of the upper lid. This may be quite bothersome. Therefore, be very careful in cutting the stitch ends from the very beginning. The stitch ends should be cut flush the knot. Next thing is to bury the knot. To do this, simply hold the stitch with a jeweler's forceps & rotate the suture. If you need to cut the stitch afterwards, the easiest process is to introduce a blade or fine needle & then just cut the suture. If any end is protruding, this can be held with a jeweler's forceps & pulled out. Otherwise this can be left within the stroma of the cornea. This will cause no harm since the 10/0 Nylon is non -irritating.

10/0 Nylon can be used for continuous suturing. The technique is very useful for cornea graft surgeries. For cataract surgery, I find interrupted suturing useful because, this can be removed should a post operative cylinder is detected. It is true that continuous suturing gives an even wound apposition & much less irritation.

If you mastered these techniques, you have become a good micro surgeon & next proceed to phaco surgery and intraocular lens implantation. I must admit that the whole field of lens implant surgery is undergoing a rapid change, newer & newer techniques, instruments, lens designs are coming. Some of the advanced techniques have been described by Dr. Mehdi Vazeen. Most important thing to realize is that, cataract surgery is not possible without becoming proficient with the microscope. Therefore, the beginner surgeon must get familiar with the different adjustments of the microscope and the operation table, adjustment of the eye piece, the IPD, Focusing control, magnification control and sitting stool. Young surgeons tend to compensate for this by extending the neck, or sitting at an uncomfortable position, as long as one can see the field, this is not desired and surgery should not be performed until the surgeon and the patient both are comfortable.

My intention is to describe the basic surgical techniques for the beginners. One can then learn the other techniques easily.

Once the beginner can learn the basics, his world is then wide open to adopt other techniques and gather higher skills. I continually modify my techniques, take up new ones & discard the previous. To a surgeon technique is important, to a patient, the result. Try to master the technique you know the best, after all, what matters is the result of your surgery. I wish to reassure you that, if you have the patience to practice the steps and master them, you can learn the most gratifying surgery in the world, cataract surgery.

**Care of the Microscope:**

Clear observation is very important at all stages. Therefore the Operating Microscope needs some care. Regularly clean the Eye Piece and the Objective lens. For countries where the humidity is high, keep a dehumidifier running in the Operation Room, because, in high humidity, Fungus grow inside the lens system and the microscope goes out of order very quickly. Microscope with good depth of focus is required. While focusing on the anterior capsule, you must be able to see the Depth of the Crater you are digging.

Standard must be maintained at the highest for all surgeries. Never perform eye surgery at a set up where you have slightest doubt that you have to compromise standard. My advice is not to compromise with two things, one is Sterilization and the other is good quality Lens and Materials

**INSTRUMENTS:**

**A. Instruments for Phaco Surgery:** Very few instruments are required for Phaco Surgery. Dr. Mehdi Vazeen suggests to use minimum instruments and to practice using the same instruments over and over again so that they virtually act as extension of surgeon's fingers. The surgeon must learn the feel, the grip and the tissue resistance with the instruments. The rationale to use minimum instruments is that by repeated use of them you will have a better feel of the instruments and how to hold and manipulate them inside the eye. The other point is, with fewer instruments, the cost is minimized and you can have more instruments trays for sterilization. The following instruments are recommended for phaco surgery:

1. Wire Speculum.
2. Fine Fixation Forceps or Fixation ring
3. Slit knife 2.5 or 2.8 mm
4. Side Port knife 15 Degree
5. Irrigating Cystitome
6. Uttarata Forceps
7. Hydrodissection Cannula attached to 5 cc syringe
8. Chopper or Sinsky Hook

9. Iris Spatula
10. Rycof's cannula attached to syringe
11. Viscoelastic filled syringe with cannula

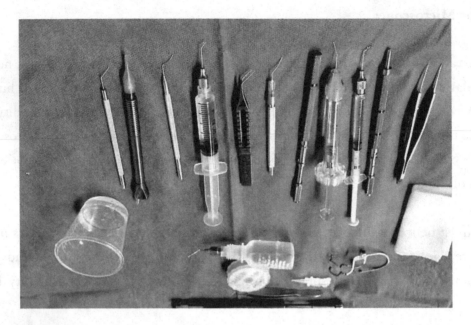

(Fig. 6 Instruments for Phacosurgery Note the number of instruments at the table. The less the number is better and easier to handle them.)

Some of these instruments are single use and should be discarded after surgery. Some of the instruments are reusable and sent for cleaning and re sterilization with autoclave or Hot Air Oven. If you have small number of instruments, it is easy to re sterilize and also inexpensive to have 4 or 5 sets ready for the number of surgeries.

Optional instrument sets may be autoclaved and kept ready should conversion become necessary during the procedure or if other accidents happen and vitrectomy and suturing become necessary. These sets can then be readily put on the tray by the nurse and be used with safety.

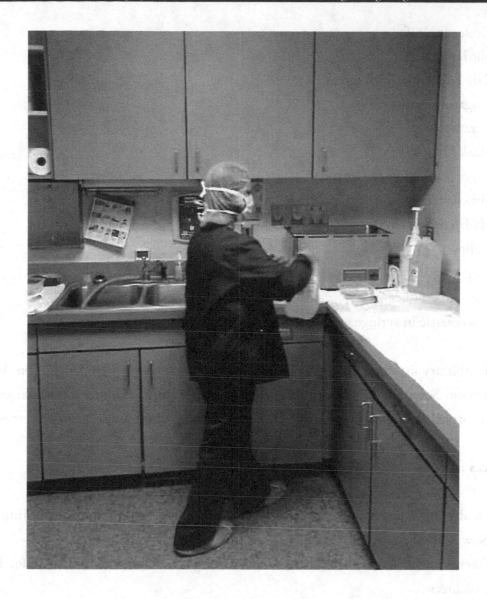

(Fig 7 : Instrument Cleaning. Note that for proper cleaning
a dedicated area and staff is required)

## B. INSTRUMENTS FOR SMALL INCISION CATARACT SURGERY (SICS) OR ECCE :

For manual SICS surgery we need few more instruments on the table. These are:

1. Wire Speculum
2. Conjunctival Scissors or Westcott Scissors.
3. Silcock's Needle Holder
4. Barraquer's Needle Holder
5. Blade Breaker with handle or Guarded Knife
6. Micro toothed forceps

7. Crescent Knife

8. Slit Knife 3.2 or 2.8

9. Side Port Knife 15 Degree

10. Irrigating cystitome

11. Utrata forceps

12. Sinsky Hook

13. Iris Spatula or Phaco Spatula

14. Simcoe Irrigating and Aspiration Cannula

15. Hydro dissection Cannula

16. Caliper

17. Irrigating Vectis

18. Capsule Polisher

19. Viscoelastic in syringe with cannula.

This is an arbitrary list of instruments required for cataract surgery. A lot depends on the liking of the surgeon. Several other instruments are used like J shaped cannula for aspiration of sub incisional cortical mater, Cautery to stop capillary bleeding. These are surgeon's discretion.

**References :**

1. Ocular microsurgery Author : LBC Ang, LCY Khoo, Arthur Lim Siew Ming,. Base : New York : Karger 1981

2. Essentials of Cataract and Lens Implant Surgery : Dr.S.M.Munirul Huq, Dr Karl Holzinger.

3. Instrumentation Guide, Ocular Surgery News Vol 6, No 11, 1995, Slack Incorporated, New Jersey, USA

4. PS Koch : Converting to Phacoemulsification Third Edition, 1992 Japee Brothers

5. Mahipal S Sachdev : Phacoemulsification A practical guide, New Age International (p) Ltd, India, Publishers 1996 P37-49

# Chapter 4
# BASIC CONCEPT OF PHACO MACHINE

Phacoemulsification is a technique of Cataract surgery which was first developed by Dr. Charles D. Kelman in 1960s is now universally used by surgeons to emulsify the cataract and remove the emulsified material by aspiration through a small incision created with a knife to enter the anterior chamber of the eye.

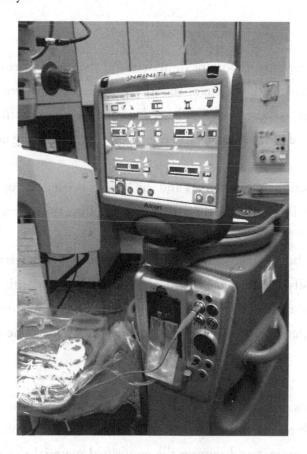

(Fig 8. The Phaco Machine: Note that there are several companies, manufacturers and models. This is one of the machines in use. Beginning surgeon needs to be proficient with the different parameter of the equipment that is being handled.)

The actual equipment is a computerized ultrasonic phacoemulsification machine in which, electrical energy is converted to mechanical energy with the help of piezo electric crystals. This ultrasound energy thus created causes the phaco tip to vibrate at a high speed, which emulsifies the lens material and the hard nucleus into tiny small particles. This emulsified material is then aspirated out of the eye using irrigation and aspiration system of the machine, which is controlled by computer programs. This tip vibration produces friction and, the mechanical friction produces heat that causes the phaco tip to become hot. The ultrasonic phacoemulsification needle is fitted with an irrigation sleeve around it. This irrigation sleeve circulates cooling fluid and carries heat away from the tip. The phaco tip with its sleeve needs to go through the incision created to enter the anterior chamber. The incision size is therefore larger than the tip diameter. In bi-manual micro phaco this problem has been resolved now by using power modulated phaco machines which keeps the phaco tip cool enough and the surgery can be performed through a much smaller incision size.

For the beginning surgeon it is important to understand the physics behind the machine and it is also easiest to learn initially. Later on, as the surgeon is more experienced and has to perform surgeries on wide variety of cataracts, will need to change the parameters and adjust them according to the structure of the eye ball and the type of cataract being addressed.

It is very difficult to describe the mechanics and the physics behind the operation of the machine but certain basic concept is required by the surgeon for handling the different parameters properly.

There are two separate but fundamental components of the phaco system. Firstly, ultrasound energy is used to emulsify the nucleus. Secondly, a fluid irrigation aspiration system is used to aspirate the emulsified material through the phaco tip or the Irrigation and aspiration hand piece of the machine. The anterior chamber depth is maintained at the same time with irrigation of fluid.

The basic question comes in mind is, which machine is the best machine for the procedure? This question is very difficult to address, all phaco machines do the same job. It produces ultrasonic power to emulsify the cataract and remove the emulsified material through the hand piece by aspiration assisted by irrigation. A basic low cost machine and a high end high cost machine both do the same job with different degrees of safety margin. My advice is, before deciding which Phaco Machine to purchase, look around, discuss with the seniors and talk to the biomedical engineer of the company who is available in your area. The sales people will definitely push to buy their machine claiming that their machine is the best, but it is the service engineers who will rescue you if things go wrong with the machine and it does not work as expected. Therefore, plan to purchase the machine from the company who has the best engineering and after sales support in your area irrespective of the price or make or model. Some companies traditionally have very good after sales service; some companies do not care about the surgeon after selling the machine. This varies from country to country, area to area and person to person. The phaco machine has developed tremendously in terms of Ultrasound power modulations and pump mechanisms in the past decade. Different manufacturers have incorporated different techniques to their machines to deliver the phaco energy with greater safety of operation. Please get familiar with the settings and the parameters of the machine before using it. Personally, I encountered machines which required complicated settings and I could not get used to them and consequently could not use the machine. The theater assistant has to understand the settings and parameters very well and requires training by the company. Ensure this before deciding to actually purchase the machine. Cleaning and maintenance of the machine is very important and one assistant has to be trained to do that. The surgeon does not have the patience or the time and energy to do this after performing the stressful surgery and completion of the sessions. The machine is very delicate and requires regular cleaning and sterilization. Learn this yourself and teach your assistant to do this properly, slightest banging or dropping of the hand piece will cause the crystals to displace and the ultrasound to malfunction.

It must be mentioned here that a basic understanding of the machine is very important for the surgeon to tame it and make the machine do what you want it to do and comprehend the nature and significance of the settings of the parameters to gain control over the equipment. Phaco surgery is a machine dependent surgery and requires highest technical skill and knowledge about the procedure.

In order to drive a car, one does not need to understand how the internal combustion gasoline engines run on a mixture of gasoline and air. The car wheels moves in a four stroke in each cylinders. The four strokes are **Intake, Compression, Power** and **Exhaust. When the air gasoline mixture reaches the cylinder, it intakes the mixture, the spark plug creates a spark and as the spark plug fires, igniting the compressed air-fuel mixture produces a powerful expansion of the vapor.** The combustion process pushes the piston down the cylinder with great force turning the crankshaft to provide the power to propel the vehicle. There are additional requirements like cooling system and Oil system, gear system, Exhaust system, Brake system, the Battery system, Emission system and the Electrical system.

We only know that, after starting the vehicle by the ignition switch and putting it in gear, pressing on the Accelerator will start propelling the vehicle in the direction we want by controlling the Steering wheel. We also know that if we want, we can stop the vehicle by pressing on the brake. The diver has to understand the basic mechanisms of running the car and the different controls.

Running and operating the phaco machine is no different but the surgeon must learn the various control mechanisms, understand when to use them and the implications of changing each parameter. It is not imperative to understand the details of how the computer processors are working inside the machine to give us what we want, the way we want it. The surgeon must know how much the foot paddle is to be depressed and when to put a brake on, or withdraw the foot to what level to stop the machine or even reverse the functions.

**Basically the Phaco Machine consists of four parts:**

1. **The Ultrasound System**: The computer processor by which electrical energy is converted into mechanical energy, the transducer converts this to ultrasound impulses which cause the tip to vibrate resulting in emulsification of the cataract.

2. **The Phaco Handpiece** is an important piece of the equipment. The ultrasound (U/S) hand piece vibrates the phaco needle at a set rate in the 20,000 to 40,000 HZ range. All the activities of the machine are translated through the hand piece which we hold and work with. It has piezo –electric crystals in it, and is attached to a needle, the Phaco tip. The Phaco tip is a titanium needle of different diameters and bends which is attached tightly to the handpiece with the help of a wrench. Tightening the tip is very important because, if loose, the tip will not vibrate properly and will not deliver the energy necessary for its function. The tip needs to be sterilized with autoclave or has to be single use. Sharpness of the tip is also important; a blunt tip will not cut as smoothly as a sharp one. The Irrigation line is attached to the handpiece which sends BSS into the eye and a separate aspiration line is attached to the handpiece which sucks the emulsified materials out of the eye. The irrigation fluid is driven to the eye which maintains the anterior chamber during these maneuvers and also cools down the phaco tip. The sleeve has to be tightly fitted to the hand piece and the exposure of the front part of the tip ensured under the microscope. Sometimes, the needle may pass through the side hole of the sleeve and cause problem during the surgery, this needs to be inspected beforehand under the microscope.

3. **The Foot Paddle**: The foot pedal is typically controlled with the dominant foot. The Foot Paddle acts like an accelerator of the car.

There are 4 positions:

Position 0 – everything is off;

Position 1 – irrigation is on, no pump, no Ultrasound;

Position 2 – irrigation is on, pump is on, and Ultrasound is off;

Position 3 – irrigation is on, pump is on, and Ultrasound is on.

As the foot paddle is depressed, the machine starts working and it is the control of the Foot Paddle is that controls the machine. Most foot paddles has a reflux mechanism so that if undesired materials are accidentally sucked in, this can be refluxed instantly by using this control.

4. **The Irrigation and Aspiration System :**

This is one of the most important computer generated systems of the machine and is more complicated to understand.

**The irrigation** system in phaco machines is typically an adjustable bottle held higher than the eye to allow infusion of fluid into the eye by the force of gravity. The irrigation tube opens by pressing on the foot paddle and opening of the pinch valve. The bottle height can be adjusted for various phases of the surgery automatically by the machine or can be done manually. The anterior chamber pressure is directly proportional to the height of the bottle. The anterior chamber depth can be altered by bottle height. This is of relevance when performing surgery on hyperopic and myopic patients. Hyperopic patients have smaller eyeball and a shallower anterior chamber. Raising the bottle height increases the depth of the anterior chamber to perform safe phacoemulsification. Myopic patients on the other hand, have longer eyeball and a deeper anterior chamber and the bottle height is lowered to get a comfortable chamber depth. Same is true in eyes with liquid vitreous where low flow is preferable.

**Irrigation /Aspiration and Vacuum settings:**

It is very important to understand the irrigation, aspiration and vacuum settings of the machine and what actually is expected of the machine at the set parameters. The surgeon has to be familiar with the effect of a 400 mm Hg vacuum vs 100 mm Hg vacuum, a 40 ml flow rate as opposed to 10 ml flow rate on the particular machine being used, whether the machine has gravity fed irrigation or a forced pump irrigation and this understanding has profound effect on the techniques of the surgery.

**Pressurized Forced Infusion Techniques**:

In phacoemulsification, ultrasound energy, vacuum and fluidic irrigation and aspiration forces work in a delicate balance to break up and remove the emulsified cataract. Fluidics depends on the infusion of balanced salt solution to maintain IOP and anterior chamber depth. Maintenance of a stable anterior chamber is very important to perform safe phaco surgery and this is difficult when the incision size is reduced as in micro- incision cataract surgery because of low flow of irrigating fluid. To address this problem, Dr. Amar Agarwal first introduced the concept of pressurized infusion and later in 2009 this was incorporated into Bausch & Lomb DigiFlow Pressurized Infusion system to the Stellaris Machine. Phaco machines use two types of infusion; passive infusion, in which gravity pulls fluid from an elevated bottle, and active or forced infusion, which is driven by gas injected into the bottle or by mechanical pumping. The Centurion Vision System (Alcon) uses a different mechanism to produce forced infusion. Instead of air being forced into the infusion bottle, a bag of balanced salt solution BSS is squeezed or relaxed by microprocessor-controlled paddles.

When the foot paddle is depressed, the irrigation is started, and when the foot paddle is further pressed, irrigation and aspiration is started and if the phaco tip is not occluded, the pump produces fluid currents in the anterior chamber due to aspiration currents which attract nuclear fragments to the tip. When a fragment completely occludes the tip, vacuum suction is activated and the pump provides holding power by vacuum suction which grips and holds the fragment. As soon as the nuclear fragment is aspirated, the vacuum falls and this causes a surge of fluid which is pulled into the tubing. In order to use the phaco machine, a surgeon must understand the different settings and the parameters of ultrasound power, vacuum, flow rate, and bottle height. This can be lowered or set higher automatically in some machines or this can be done manually and the fluid stand is marked in Centimeters for this purpose.

The irrigation aspiration system of the phaco machines work through a pump mechanism. There are three types of Pumps:

- Peristaltic Pumps
- Venturi Pumps
- Hybrid Pumps

Different companies employ the different pumps to create vacuum for aspiration of the emulsified material and cortical mater from the eye.

### A. Peristaltic Pumps :

Peristaltic pump acts on the principle of peristalsis or propagating the fluid along a line through a flexible tube. The fluid is propagated along the tube by a rotating circular drum which has rollers or shoes attached on the outer side of the drum. The number of rollers has to be more than two. When the rotor moves, the tube is pinched and is closed forcing the fluid forward by creating vacuum in the tube. The tube opens to drain the fluid out of the pump. Peristaltic pump can run continuously or may work intermittently causing partial revolutions to control the creation of vacuum. However, how quickly the preset level will be raised is programmed on to the machine and is called the rise time. As the vacuum rises, the rollers slow down and pressure builds up and ultimately the rollers stop when the preset vacuum is reached.

In peristaltic pumps one needs to set up the irrigation rate expressed in cc per minute and aspiration vacuum expressed in mm Hg.

### B. Venturi Pump System:
The vacuum in venturi machine is created by using the principle of venturi effect to create a vacuum. The Venturi effect is the reduction in fluid pressure that results when a fluid flows through a constricted section of pipe. The vacuum level is created within a rigid drainage cassette system, to which the phaco aspiration tubing is connected. The venturi pump is able to create the preset vacuum level without occlusion of the phaco tip. When the surgeon depresses the foot pedal, the preset vacuum level is immediately created with or without occlusion. Thus the cataract is removed quicker in venturi machines. It is named after the Italian Scientist, Giovanni Battista Venturi.

### C. Hybrid Pumps:
These pumps can act like a peristaltic pump or a venturi pump depending upon the programming. This type of pumps are recent additions to the pump systems and with the advantage of both types of pumps, the surgeon can decide which type of operation of the machine is required at which stage of the surgery. All modern phaco machines incorporate both the principles of pump systems controlled by computer chips and manipulated by the surgeon to the advantage of the surgical procedure.

**SURGE :**

Surge occurs when the phaco tip is occluded by the fragment and is held by high vacuum which rises to the preset level if occlusion is maintained. Emulsification of the fragment clears the occlusion and the emulsified material is abruptly aspirated. The tubing expands on breaking of the occlusion by aspiration of the fragment which was occluding the tip. This causes a rush of fluid from the anterior chamber into the phaco tip to equilibrate the buildup of vacuum in the aspiration line. If the fluid in the anterior chamber is not replaced rapidly enough by the irrigation line, the anterior chamber becomes shallow with a rapid anterior movement of the posterior capsule. This may cause posterior capsule rupture along with other complications. The surge can be modified by selecting lower levels of vacuum and adjusting the flow rate. In addition to these preventive measures, phaco machines use a variety of methods to combat surge. Surge cannot be fully abolished and it is up to the surgeon to be alert during surgery to prevent sudden aspiration of fragments during chopping and other maneuvers. Although the newer machines has developed technology to combat and reduce the surge such as the Centurion Vision System phaco machine by Alcon that works by continually monitoring the anterior chamber for Intraocular Pressure stabilization and thus abolishes surge, the surgeon should understand the mechanism of surge and prevent this during surgery.

1.  **AMO Sovereign and Alcon Infinity:** These machines use a microprocessor to sample vacuum and flow parameters 50 times per second. As soon as surge is sensed by the sensor, the machine computer slows and reverses the pump in order to stop surge production.

2.  **Bausch & Lomb Millennium:** These machines use dual linear foot Paddle control which separates flow and vacuum. The emulsification occurs in the presence of a lower vacuum and surge is minimized.

3.  **Alcon Infinity and Alcon Legacy:** these machines use Aspiration Bypass System (ABS) to minimize surge, which do not abolish but dampens the surge on occlusion break.

4.  **Preocclusion Phaco, Neosonic X technology of Alcon:** These machines use Micropulse phaco to abolish occlusion and therefore surge and vacuum are not allowed to build up. This allows fragment removal with minimum energy level and in a deep and controlled anterior chamber.

5.  **Centurion Phaco System :** The new Centurion Vision System phaco machine of ALCON uses active stable pressure in the anterior camber to prevent surge by continuous intraocular pressure monitoring and stabilization.

**Phaco Power Generation :**

It is important to have an understanding about how the phaco machines generate power for emulsification of the hard nucleus of the cataract, because, use of the generated power has to be judicious for optimum surgical result. Little power will scratch on the surface of the nucleus. Too much power will cause wound burn and corneal damage leading to complications.

Phaco machine has a computer to generate ultrasonic impulses which then pass on to the Hand Piece. There are Piezo- electric Crystals in the handpiece which converts these electrical impulses to mechanical energy. The mechanical energy thus produced causes the Titanium needle to vibrate at a very high speed. The ultrasound energy vibrates the phaco tip at a set rate between 20,000 to 45,000 Hz (cycles per second) range. Most hand pieces have four piezo electric crystals. Increasing the Ultrasound power increases the excursion of the needle but not the frequency which remains stable.

Before starting the surgery, the phaco hand piece has to be tuned. During" tuning" the machine sends pulse to the hand piece and sees how much power must be delivered to move the needle in the particular medium. Tuning of the hand piece and the machine is important because, the phaco tip has to operate in different media and small alterations in the frequency are created to operate in the different media by "tuning" the circuitry in the computer.

The Nucleus of the cataract is harder than the cortex and this is emulsified by several forces generated by movement of the needle.

1.  Jack Hammer effect
2.  Cavitations
3.  Acoustic shock effect
4.  Impact of the fluid particle wave

Stroke length is the length of the movement of the needle which is generally 2 to 6 mills (one thousandth of an inch); longer stroke length will create excess heat.

**Jack Hammer Effect:**

When Phaco energy is applied, the "phaco tip vibrates at ultrasonic speed in a longitudinal direction. This causes the needle to produce physical striking force of the needle against the nucleus. It is thought that this physical striking force causes the nucleus to be emulsified.

**Cavitations:**

The Phaco tip is a needle which due to the movement at ultrasonic speed in the aqueous creates intense zones of high and low pressures.

Low pressure is created by the backward movement of the phaco tip produces micro bubbles. High pressure created by forward movement of the phaco tip produces compression of the micro bubble until they burst inwards causing an intense shock wave of about 75,000 PSI. This shock wave is very powerful and radiates from the phaco tip in the direction of the bevel of the tip. The transient cavitations are a violent event that lasts for 6 to 256 milliseconds. These transient cavitations may be responsible to generate the energy for emulsification of the hard material of the nucleus.

**The Phaco machine can be set up at a variety of ultrasound modes:**

Continuous mode, Pulse Mode, Burst Mode and Hyper pulse Mode.

**Continuous Mode:** In continuous mode, the U/S is on when the foot paddle is depressed in position 3 and increases in intensity or power the deeper the surgeon goes in position 3 up to a set maximum.

**Pulse Mode:** The ultrasound in pulse mode is a basic type of power modulation that relies on alternating phaco-on time with phaco-off time. Each shot of ultrasound energy is referred to as a pulse. The surgeon is able to control the power delivered via foot pedal at position 3. The power will be delivered in pulses up to a pre set maximum then there is a period of no ultrasound. A

50 % duty cycle is common setting. A Duty cycle is the ratio of phaco-on time to total (or cycle) time, expressed as a percentage. In other words, phaco-on time / (phaco-on time + phaco-off time). Setting power modulation at one pulse per second with a 50 percent duty cycle would give 500 ms phaco-on + 500 ms phaco-off.

**Burst mode:** In this mode, a burst of phaco power is delivered and a duty cycle is chosen. After setting the burst duration from 80 to 600 ms, depression of the foot pedal in position 3 allows linear control of the duty cycle between this minimum and maximum. The further the foot paddle is depressed in position 3, the shorter the phaco-off time. If the maximum duty cycle is set at 100 percent, then with maximum foot depression ultrasound delivery becomes continuous.

**Hyper pulse mode:** allows the surgeon to choose higher-range pulse settings that can be 100 pulses per second as opposed to 20 pulses per second in standard pulse mode. Each short phaco pulse is followed by a short phaco-off time. This does not cause more amount of phaco energy used by using more pulses per second, the off period reduces the energy delivered at each cycle.

**Tortional Hand piece:**

Some phaco machines have come up with tortional handpiece. In additional to the classical linear longitudinal movement, these hand pieces incorporate a tortional component. AMO has an 8 motion handpiece; Alcon OZIL has a rotational feature. The advantage is that, the phaco energy when applied do not push the nucleus, rather the nuclear fragments come to the phaco tip easily. This tip maintains occlusion which facilitates vacuum build-up and reduces flow through the anterior chamber decreasing turbulence, therefore reducing the likelihood of lens particles damaging the corneal endothelial cells.

**Parameters setting at different stages of the surgery:** This depends upon the type of cataract being addressed, the stage of the surgery and the technique being performed by the surgeon and the machine being used. For a moderately hard cataract, for a machine with a peristaltic pump sculpting requires more energy and fewer vacuums and enough flow rate to cool the phaco tip. The phaco tip should cut through the cataract without rocking or pushing the nucleus and putting stress on the zonules. Thus, a 60 to 80 % Phaco power, 80 mm Hg vacuum and 20 cc per minute flow rate should be optimal.

When chopping, the fragments need to be held firmly and higher vacuum higher flow rate and lower ultrasound energy is required. Thus, a 300 mm Hg vacuum, 30 cc flow rate and 40 to 50%

phaco power should be adequate to hold and chop the nucleus. In venturi pumps or vacuum pumps, the settings will be different.

The parameters in the modern power modulated machines require different settings and this must be learned well before operating the machine. The other important thing is to use the parameters judiciously so that the intended functions are carried out by the machine. During sculpting, low power will only scratch on the surface of the nucleus without actually cutting it and high vacuum will hold the nucleus firmly but will not cut it.

On the other hand, high vacuum will hold the nucleus firmly for chopping but in order to get a firm grip, the phaco tip needs to be buried into the nucleus using phaco energy and full vacuum rise to preset level will only happen when the tip is fully occluded.

Thus, using power and aspiration flow rate at the appropriate step and at appropriate level will give good surgical result.

It is to be noted that, the phaco machine is an extension of the brain of the surgeon and the instruments are extension of the fingers and every occurrences inside the eye during surgery is related to some principles of Physics. It is important to understand the physics of the steps, the vectors, the forces and so on. If this can be appreciated by the surgeon, then the importance of the excursion of the instruments inside the eye, the amount of suction to be applied or ultrasound required for cutting and emulsification can be appreciated. Therefore, the surgeon should familiarize with the machine parameters and understand what they mean in terms of settings and output at every step of the surgery keeping in mind that, different machines operate differently.

A good driver should have full knowledge of driving as well as be able to understand some mechanics to figure out whether the car is running smoothly. Thus, the surgeon must know the machine parameters for smooth functioning of the machine at every step of the surgery. Simple knowledge about the basic mechanisms of phaco machine will enable the surgeon to perform safer surgery. It is a true blend of technology and technique. The surgeon should be able to modify parameters as needed during the surgery of a particular cataract at a particular situation. A skilful surgeon with knowledge of the principles of the machine is in a better position to understand the parameters and obtain better results of the surgery. Modern phaco machines are designed with high level of safety and control. Thus careful attention, with technique designed to optimize the machine's performance, will result in the safest, most efficient phacoemulsification surgery.

## REFERENCES:

1  Hoffman, R. S. et al. Curr Opin Ophthalmol 2005;16:38-43.

2  Fishkind, W. et al. J Cataract Refract Surg 2006;32:45-49.

3  Seibel, B. S. Phacodynamics: Mastering the Tools and Techniques of Phacoemulsification Surgery, 4th Edition (Thorofare, N.J.: Slack Inc., 2005), 114-125.

4  Devgan, U. Ophthalmol Clin North Am 2006;19(4):457-468

5  Understanding the fundamentals of Power Modulation in Phacoemulsification :Graham W. Lyles, Kenneth L. Cohen MD

6  Fishkind WJ Neuhann TF, Steinert RF. The phaco Machine, in Cataract Surgery, Technique Complications & Management. Chapter 6, second Edition, Philadelphia, PA : WB Saunders, 2004 PP 61-77

7  Vasavada, A.R.,et al. Comparison of torsional and microburst longitudinal phacoemulsification: a prospective, randomized, masked clinical trial. Ophthalmic Surg Lasers Imaging, 2010. 41(1): p. 109-14.

# Chapter 5

# PATIENT SELECTION AND INVESTIGATIONS

Patient selection plays an important role in successful cataract surgery. The surgeon must understand the type, maturity of cataract, location of the opacity and the type of surgery required for the individual patient.

The crystalline Lens is a biconvex, avascular, transparent structure enclosed by a capsule, which is the basement membrane secreted by the lens epithelium. A ring of zonular fibers, inserting on the ciliary body suspends the lens to the ciliary body.

Any opacity whether congenital or acquired in the lens capsule, cortex, nucleus or substance of the lens, irrespective of its effect on vision is called cataract.

**Classification of cataract:**
   A. Congenital Cataract
   B. Age related Cataract
   C. Secondary Cataract
   D. Cataract in systemic Disease.

**Classification of Age related Cataract:**

   1. Anterior polar and subcapsular cataract
   2. Posterior Subcapsular Cataract
   3. Nuclear Cataract
   4. Cortical Cataract
   5. Total Cataract

**Secondary Cataract:**

1. Cataract in anterior uveitis
2. Cataract in Ac. Congestive Glaucoma
3. Cataract in Myopia
4. Cataract in Hereditary Fundus Dystrophy, e.g., Retinitis Pigmentosa
5. Cataract in Systemic Disease :
6. Diabetes Mellitus
7. Myotonic Dystrophy
8. Atopic Dermatitis
9. Neurofibromatosis.

**Cataract according to maturity:**

1. Immature Cataract
2. Mature Cataract
3. Hypermature Cataract
4. Morgagnian Cataract

**Grading of Nucleus according to Hardness:**

Clinically, hardness of the nucleus is examined on the slit lamp for grading. The grading is important because, this gives a guide to the ease of performing phaco surgery and the decision for employing the techniques for the surgery.

**Grade 0: Soft Nucleus**

Grade 1: White or Greenish yellow Color Nucleus

Grade 2: Yellow colored Nucleus: Moderately hard

Grade 3: Amber Colored Nucleus: Hard nucleus

Grade 4: Brown or Black Colored Nucleus: Very hard in consistency

Grade 5: Milky white cataract: Very hard Nucleus with liquid cortex.

This is an arbitrary classification, and grading, the surgeon may make his own classification of hardness of the nucleus as the nucleus is examined in a dilated patient on the slit lamp.

Phacoemulsification is the state of the art in cataract surgery and is developing very rapidly in instrumentation, technique and concept. The ophthalmologist learns one technique in cataract surgery uses one machine and within a short period of time, a new machine and technology becomes available, the old machine is outdated and new machine is to be purchased. In spite of this fact, the satisfaction the surgeon gets in serving the patient with the latest technology outcasts the struggle.

Phaco surgery is not the only procedure in cataract surgery, if properly performed, other techniques like SICS or ECCE with PC IOL implant also gives equally or near equal surgical outcome. The surgeon has to decide which technique is to be adopted for which patient. The technique is important to the surgeon, the result to the patient.

Phacoemulsification is possible in all types of cataract but the amount of energy to be employed to emulsify the hard cataract may be so much that, it may cause damage to the corneal endothelium and or damage to the posterior capsule. Therefore, one has to decide to choose the surgical technique to be used on a particular form of cataract in a particular patient. The beginners should perform phaco surgeries on Grade 0 to 3 types of cataract. Plan Small Incision Cataract Surgery (SICS) for the other types of nucleus and in hyper mature milky white cataracts and morgagnian cataracts.

## PREOPERATIVE INVESTIGATIONS:

Some preoperative investigations are to be performed before cataract surgery for the safety of the patient and the surgeon.

### History:

A full history including existing medical disease like diabetes, hypertension, bronchial asthma, IHD, prostatic hypertrophy, bleeding disorders, mental illness. History of using all medicines used by the patient specially the use of medications including anticoagulation agents, Flomax for prostate, Nitroglycerin for angina or Salbutamol spray for Asthma.

Present or past dental infections, drug allergy, trauma, ocular inflammation or any past ocular disease.

## Systemic Investigations:

1. Blood Pressure: Control of Systemic Hypertension is a must before cataract surgery
2. Blood Sugar: Adequate control of Glycemic status is important and is to be tested.
3. Urine for Examination: Routine and Microscopic examination of the urine particularly albumin, sugar and pus cells.
4. Resting Electro Cardiogram to exclude any active cardiac problems.
5. Dental Check up in selected cases
6. Conjunctival Swab for culture and sensitivity if any infection is anticipated
7. Patency of the Nasolacrimal system

## Ocular Investigations:

1. Visual Acuity. If V/A is not recordable, Finger count, Perception of light and Projection of rays
2. Pupil: Pupillary response to light
3. Slit lamp examination: Before and after dilatation of the pupil, Intraocular Pressure
4. Fundus examination: by Direct and Indirect Ophthalmoscope
5. Estimation of post operative visual acuity: by PAM or other methods.
6. Macular Function tests: To evaluate macula the following tests can be performed:

   a) Two point discrimination test
   b) Maddox Rod Test
   c) Color Vision test
   d) Worth's Four Dot Test
   e) Pupillary Light reflex test
   F) Illuminated Amsler Grid
   g) Macular Photo stress test

**Please refer to sample workout sheet of Dr. Mehdi Vazeen in Appendix**

**BIOMETRY:** Biometry involves calculation of the power of the IOL to be implanted. This can be done in the following ways:

## 1. **Based on the previous refraction and glasses used.**

When the ultrasound A scan to measure the axial length of the eye ball was not available, this was an approximate method of calculating the power of the IOL to be implanted. This rough estimate can be used where A scan is not available.

First, previous refraction before cataract formation is found out from previous records, and where not available, we used to do lensometry on the previous spectacle to find out the dioptric value of the Glass. This can also be done by Neutralizing method.

**Formula for the IOL power calculation is : P = 19 D + (R X 1.25)**
**P= The power of IOL, R = The previous refraction power of glasses in Dioptre.**
**Example, a patient with – 3.00 myopia will require:**
**P = 19 D + (-3 X 1.25) = 15.25 D (approximate power of the IOL)**

## 2, **Using SRK formula:**

**P = A – 2.5 X L -0.9X K**
**P= Power of IOL, A = A constant for the particular lens, K = Keratometry reading, L= Axial length measured by A scan biometry.**

## 3. **Using Theoretical formulas :**

**These formulae have superseded the regression formulae. There are three commonly used third-generation theoretical formulae are:**

    a.  **The SRK-T**
    b.  **Holladay-1**
    c.  **Hoffer Q.**

**Keratometry :**

    1)  **Manual Keratometer :** B& L type : used to measure Keratometry and recorded
    2)  **Auto Keratometer :** Used to document Keratometry readings and recorded

**Axial Length Measurement :**

a) Ultrasound A scan for measuring the axial length of the eye.

b) Immersion biometry

c) Partial coherence interferometery biometry is a new non-invasive method for measuring The axial length.

## THE IOL MASTER:

The lOL Master is a device that uses partial coherent interferometery to measure axial length. It has a number of possible advantages over traditional ultrasound methods in that it does not require contact with the cornea, has additional facilities to measure corneal curvature and also has a higher resolution. The disadvantage is that this cannot be done in very Mature and Hypermature cataracts.

**Biometry in intumescent and calcified cataract:**

Waterlogged and intumescent lenses dampen the sound velocity. This would lead to using an axial length that is 0.15 mm longer than it should be, resulting in about +/-0.5 D error in the final refraction.

Calcified cataract causes total reflection of the sound waves and as a result no retinal spike is recorded in the A-scan.

The clinician may have to choose the intraocular lens implant (IOL) power according to the refractive history or else could use the axial length from the other eye. This will result in approximate power as described earlier.

**IOL power calculation after Refractive surgery**

More and more patients with cataracts who have a history of refractive surgery are coming for cataract surgery and their Intraocular Power Calculation is more complex. It is better if a prior Biometry is obtained for these patients before Refractive corrections had been done. Modern methods give an adequate IOL power calculation for these patients.

**Biometry after trabeculectomy**

Axial length measurement may decrease after a successful trabeculectomy operation. Biometry in phakic eyes with a history of trabeculectomy may result in wrong postoperative refractive results.

Measurement of axial length before the trabeculectomy operations is recommended.

**The following are some points to be noted during pre operative assessment:**

1. Discussions regarding full procedure and possible outcome and complications, which type of anesthesia is to be used and which type of lens will be implanted are important considerations.

2. Full eye examination with Slit Lamp is essential.
   Note any eye lid diseases like Blepharitis, Stye or Dry Eye Syndrome, Conjunctiva Scarring, Corneal thickness and Endothelium, Iris and Pupillary regularity and response to light. Next examine the Nucleus note the type of cataract and dilate the pupil.

3. Note the dilation, Posterior synechiae, Anterior capsule, Cortical plaques, Hardness of the Nucleus and the Posterior capsule. Extent and ease of dilatation is to be noted, in Diabetics, Glaucoma or Iritis, Pupil dilates slowly.

4. Cataract in one eye requires special attention and in these cases, elucidate any history of trauma, if present look for integrity of the Zonules and get an Ultrasound B scan if necessary.

5. Measure the Intraocular Pressure and patency of the Lachrymal Sac or if there is any regurgitation present on pressure on the sac area.

6. Check the condition of the Macula by Macular function tests, Ophthalmoscopy, OCT or PAM (Potential Acuity Meter): I have been caught on occasions with Macular Scar or Macular Hole after cataract surgery.

7. Get an ECG, Blood Sugar, Blood pressure and Chest X ray. Conjunctival Swab Culture is performed by many surgeons, but I think not contributory.

8. If the patient is diabetic, control of Blood sugar is important and also examination of the Fundus by indirect Ophthalmoscopy.

9. **Perform Biometry to find out the Power of the Lens to be implanted.**

If there is a preexisting medical or surgical condition, for example, uncontrolled Diabetes, Hypertension, Ischemic heart disease, Enlargement of Prostate, Back or spinal problems, appropriate Physician or Surgeon must be consulted and permission obtained regarding the precautions to be taken during and after surgery. If the patient is receiving any medication for Prostate, stop three days before surgery and also be mentally prepared for Floppy Iris syndrome.

Do not Applanate the cornea just before the surgery, for Tonomertry or for Biometry as this may reduce clarity of the cornea during surgery. At least three days must pass before you plan for surgical date and such eye examination.

Preoperatively I use topical antibiotic drops six times a day for at least two days. If culture report is available, appropriate drops or Ciprofloxacin drops and NSAID Drop is used three times a day for two days. Many surgeons prefer to give one tab. Acetazolamide and one tab Diazepam before surgery to alleviate anxiety.

The patient is given the date and time to report for surgery. The Intraocular Lens to be implanted along with Biometry report must be recorded and a copy kept with the records at the center. I found many patients reporting for surgery without the Biometry report and if no records are available; this has to be repeated causing delay and disappointments.

**Day of the Surgery**

Cataract Surgery is Day Case surgery and do not need hospitalization. The patients are advised to come on the day of the surgery. A complete and step by step preparation is therefore required for smooth functioning of the surgical plan. Many times due to hurry, the patient may be sent to the Operation Room without a Consent form signed and this may cause endless trouble to the surgeon.

After the patient arrives for surgery to the surgery center, three things are very important:

1. Obtain Informed consent of the patient, signed by the patient or next of Keen, always witnessed by at least two other persons is most important.
2. A history sheet with all the findings must be noted by an assistant.
3. Face wash and clean dress, possibly one supplied by the hospital, preferably autoclaved patient gown.

## PUPIL DILATATION :

Full dilatation of the pupil is a must in order to perform Phaco Surgery. To dilate the pupil several agents are used. Tropicamide 1% eye drops, Cyclopentolate 1% eye drops, Phenylephrine 2.5 % eye drops are commonly used. Cyclopentolate is potent dilating drop but it is also long acting. I prefer to use a combination of Tropicamide 1% and Phenylephrine 2.5 % eye drops every 5 minutes for half an hour before surgery.

NSAID drops and Ciprofloxacin eye drops every 10 minutes are installed for the same period.

After the patient arrives, one or two drops topical anesthetic (tetracaine, proparacaine, etc.) instilled into the inferior conjunctival fornix.

A cotton ball, soaked in the drops can be placed into the inferior conjunctival fornix and kept there for half an hour. A dilated pupil is obtained after about 30 minutes. This avoids the necessity of application of multiple drops. Once in the operating room, the cotton ball is removed and discarded.

One drop povidone Iodine is instilled in the conjunctival sac. The lids are cleaned with 10% povidone Iodine and further cleaned with Chlorhexidine.

The patient lies on the operation table comfortably in supine position and the head should be supported. Some patients may not be able to lie flat due to kyphosis or cervical spondylitis and they should be made comfortable using higher head rest, or pillows under the buttocks. One must take into consideration that the patient has to lie still for a period of about half an hour facing the microscope and it is very distressing if full comfort is not ascertained from the very start. A sterile drape is applied after the cardiac monitor and Pulse Oximeter are attached. Comfort in breathing and position of the drape should be checked at the same time.

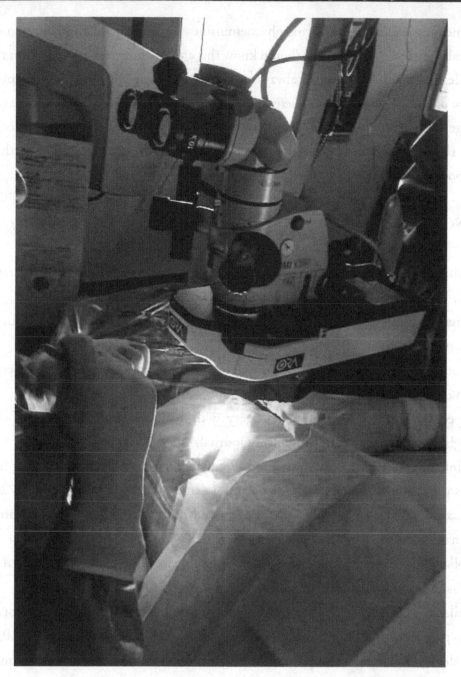

(Fig. 9 Draped patient under the Microscope: Note that proper
draping is required no area can remain uncovered. In the figure the
patient is fully draped including a sticky patch over the eye.)

The patient should be given the instructions in clear language about what to expect during surgery
and the importance of lying quietly is to be emphasized. The microscope light is a very strong
light and may be distressing for some patients. The patient must be briefed about the dangers of
sudden movement of the head, sitting up or movement of the body during surgery. The patient

will feel some pressure in the eye during phacoemulsification and during implantation of the lens under topical anesthesia. The patients should know this and the surgeon should inform the patient before the desired manipulation. It is always very desirable to say a few words of encouragement and keep the operation theatre atmosphere soothing. The patient is conscious and hears everything during surgery, therefore inappropriate remarks, jokes or any sound that may be distressing to the patient should be avoided. Once the surgery is finished, the patient should be thanked for excellent cooperation.

## REFERENCES :

1.  Mahipal S Sachdev : Phacoemulsification A practical guide, New Age International (p) Ltd, India, Publishers 1996,Applied anatomy of the lens

2.  Samar K. Basak,: Essentials of Ophthalmology, Chapter 15 pp 182 -200, Current Book International, Jan 2004

3.  Aramberri J. Intraocular lens power calculation after corneal refractive surgery: Double K method. J Cataract Refract Surg.3;29:2063-8.

4.  Boyed BF. Undergoing cataract surgery with a master surgeon: personal experience. Highlights of Ophthalm. Bi-monthly Journal, 1999; 27 (1);3

5.  Grinbaum A, Treister G, Moisseiev J. Predicted and actual refraction after intraocular lens implantation in eyes with silicone oil. J Cataract Refract Surg 1996;22:726-9.

6.  Grusha YO, Masket S, Miller KM. Phacoemulsification and lens implantation after pars plana vitrectomy. Ophthalmology. 1998;105:287-94.

7.  Holladay JT. Intraocular lens power in difficult cases. In: Masket S, Crandal AS (Eds). Atlas of Cataract Surgery. London: Martin Dunitz; 1999; 14

8.  Holladay JT, Gills JP, Leidlein J, et al. Achieving emmetropia in extremely short eyes with two piggyback posterior chamber intraocular lenses. Ophthalmology. 1996;103:1118-23,

9.  Hoffer KJ. Intraocular lens power calculation for eyes after refractive keratotomy. J Refract Surg. 1995;! 1:490-3.

10. Hoffer KJ. The Hoffer Q formula: a comparison of theoretic and regression formulas. J Cataract Surg. 1993;19:700-12.

11. Hoffer KJ. Ultrasound velocities for axial eye length measurement. J Cat Refract Surg. 1994;20:554-62.

12. Lyle WA, Jin GJ. Intraocular lens power prediction in patients who undergo cataract surgery following previous radial keratotomy. Arch Ophthalmol. 1997;! 15:457-61.

13. Maeda N, Klyce SD, Smolek MK, et al. Disparity between keratometry-style reading and corneal power within the pupil after refractive surgery for myopia. Cornea. 1997;16:517-24.

14. McCartney DL, Miller KM, Stark WJ, et al. Intraocular lens style and refraction in eyes treated with silicone oil. Arch Ophthalmol. 1987;105:1385-7.

15. Olsen T, Thim K, Corydon L. Theoretical versus SRK I and SRKII calculation of intraocular lens power. J Cataract Refract Surg. 1990;16:217-25.

16. Sanders DR, Retzlaff J, Kraff MC, et al. Comparison of the SRK/T formula and other theoretical and regression formulas. J Cataract Refract Surg. 1990; 16(3): 341-6.Pp 12-15, New Age International (p) Limited 1996

# Chapter 6
# OCULAR ANESTHESIA

Some form of Anesthesia is required for successful cataract surgery. The type of anesthesia instituted depends upon several factors.

1) How long the surgery is expected
2) What is the psychological makeup of the patient
3) Age of the Patient
4) Cooperation of the patient
5) Preference of the surgeon.
   - I recommend regional local anesthesia with light sedation for the beginners who expect the surgical time will be more than 45 minutes.
   - If the surgeon is proficient and the nucleus is up to Grade 3, and surgical time is expected to be less than 30 minutes, Topical anesthesia with light sedation is preferred.
   - Any Nucleus from Grade 4 to Grade 5, I prefer regional anesthesia.
   - If the Patient is not able to cooperate or follow surgeons command, use Regional anesthesia
   - If the patient is a child below 15 years, General anesthesia

**REGIONAL LOCAL ANESTHESIA:**

During the time when we used to perform Intracapsular Extraction of Cataract through a big 12 mm limbal wound, full akinesia and anesthesia including sedation of the patient was very important. Because, slightest squeeze of the eye would push the vitreous and contents of the eyeball out of the big open wound.

**The following are the forms of regional anesthesia commonly applied:**

Anesthetic agents: A cocktail of Xylocaine 2% and Bupivacaine 0.5 % in equal quantities mixed with Hyaluronidase is prepared and taken in a 10 CC syringe or a 5 cc syringe.

## BLOCKING THE FACIAL NERVE

**A. O' Brian's Technique**: Usually 5 ML of the mixture of the Local anesthetic prepared is injected near the Periosteum of the Neck of the mandible. The site of the Neck of the mandible is predetermined by opening and closing the Jaw of the patient. Gentle massage is applied and the whole Facial nerve is blocked including the Orbicularis Oculi.

**B. Van Lint's Method**: The Local anesthetic is injected across the branches of the Facial nerve as they pass over the Zygomatic bone. A 5 CM 25 G needle is taken and 5 CC local anesthetic is injected in the desired position around the zygomatic bone. Massage over the injection site is applied. This blocks all the motor branches of the Facial Nerve.

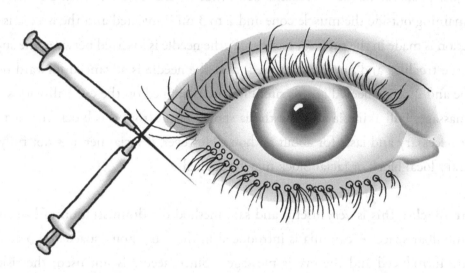

(Fig.10: Blocking the Facial Nerve : Van Lint's Method Note
that this one of the ways to block the facial nerve.)

**C. Atkinson Block** : In this method, the needle enters at the lateral border of the orbital rim at the inferior border of the Zygomatic bone and 5 CC injection is given at this site.

**D. Spaeth block**: The injection is made into the back of the mandibular condyle, just below the ear, catching the Facial Nerve as it divides.

## CILIARY BLOCK:

**Retrobulbar Block**: This is the longest practiced local anesthesia for more than 100 years. A retrobulbar needle (27 G) is fitted on to the syringe with 5 CC of the anesthetic agent prepared. The needle is passed through the skin of the lower lid at the junction of medial two third and lateral one third of the inferior orbital margin which is 5 mm medial to lateral canthus and is inserted parallel to the Optic nerve and passed through the muscle cone to the ciliary ganglion 3 to 4 CC of anesthetic is injected in the Retrobulbar space. The eye is massaged or a Super Pinky is applied for five minutes before surgery.

**Paribulbar Block**: Paribulbar anesthesia is superior to Retrobulbar injection for the reason of safety and is less painful. The same anesthetic solution **2% Lidocaine** and 0.5 % **Bupivacaine** mixture is taken in a 5 cc syringe or a 10 cc syringe. The syringe is fitted with a 23G semi blunt needle. Firstly, a small amount of solution is injected to the skin at the junction of medial two third and lateral one third of the inferior orbital margin, the needle is then advanced and 1 ml is injected just posterior to the orbicularis oculi muscle, the needle is then advanced past the equator remaining outside the muscle cone and 2 to 3 ml is injected and the needle is removed. Next, injection is made in the superior nasal area. The needle is inserted between the supraorbital notch and the trochlea and one cc is injected, next the needle is advanced forward outside the muscle cone and 2 cc is injected at this site. Pressure is applied on the eye ball with super pinki or digital massage. Full akinesia and anesthesia should result from this block and facial block is usually not necessary and lasts for about an hour. However, if facial nerve is not fully blocked, supplementary local block or facial block may be applied.

**Parabulbar Block** : This is very useful and safe method of administration of local anesthesia to the Retrobulbar space. A cannula is introduced in the sub tenon's space and 3 cc anesthetic mixtures are introduced and the eye is messaged. Since needle is not used, the risk of globe perforation is abolished.

**Topical anesthesia:**

Topical anesthesia is the preferred form of anesthesia for majority of cataract patients who are cooperative and able to follow surgeons command. The advantages of topical anesthesia are too many, but prompt visual rehabilitation and no risk of globe perforation are the most important ones. Three forms of topical anesthesia are practiced.

**1. Topical anesthetic drops only:**

In most cases installation of tetracaine or propacaine every three to four minutes six to eight times before draping and four times after the patient is draped and betadine washed away, gives adequate anesthesia. Installation of local anesthetic jelly serves the same purpose. The patient will feel pressure during viscoelastic introduction and during introduction of the IOL and they have to be alerted regarding this beforehand. In some patients low dose intravenous Fentinyl or other forms of sedation is necessary to alleviate anxiety. Presence of an anesthetist is essential to put the patient in sleep should this be required and airway monitored during the procedure. The surgeon should avoid manipulation of conjunctiva and iris during surgery which is painful. Should a complication like posterior capsule tear and vitreous loss occur, the surgeon should promptly give regional facial nerve block in Van Lint method and give small amount of Paribulbar anesthesia. This combined with sedation gives enough safety for the additional surgical time required for management of the situation.

## 2. Topical Anesthesia with Intracameral injection:

Topical anesthetic drops like tetracaine is installed in the conjunctival sac three times before draping. The eye speculum is placed and a side port incision is made using a 15 degree knife at the desired point. A ring or forceps is used to stabilize the eye and to give counter pressure on the cornea, opposite the site of entry. Grasping the conjunctiva with forceps is painful and is to be avoided. Little amount of aqueous is allowed to escape. A 2 ml syringe is filled with 1% non preserved Xylocaine and a cannula is fitted. A small amount, usually 0.5 ml of the Xylocaine is irrigated into the anterior chamber through the paracentesis and one drop is placed on the cornea. This gives adequate anesthesia and the patient is usually comfortable throughout surgery. However, they need to be instructed to keep the eyes open and fix at the microscope light and may require mild sedation to alleviate anxiety.

## 3. Topical anesthesia with van lint block:

Some patients are unable to open the eye lids and keep on squeezing the eye in the presence of microscope light and keep on moving the head. In these cases, a facial nerve block in the van lint method and Topical anesthesia with intracameral irrigation of Xylocaine gives adequate anesthesia required for the surgery.

If the patient is still not comfortable, and is non cooperative, Parabulbar injection of 2 ml Xylocaine 2% is usually enough to give the required analgesia and akinesia for the surgery. A Parabulbar infiltration of 2 ml local anesthetic with a cannula through a conjunctival incision into the subtenon's space also gives good local anesthesia and akinesia. This may be augmented with systemic sedatives like Fentinyl or Midazolam HCL 1 ml by the anesthetist.

**Sedation and Monitoring for Cataract Surgery:**

Some patients do not require sedation and the presence of an anesthetist to monitor the vital signs during surgery is important.

For many patients surgery on their eyes causes anxiety. The fear of losing one's sight can be overwhelming. Sedation can decrease anxiety, thereby increasing cooperation during surgery. Patient's perception of surgery at completion is of a few pleasant moments that took place during the procedure.

Medication for sedation can be: 1) Oral agents, 2) Intramuscular agents 3) IV sedation

**Oral Medication for adults:**

a)  Versed (Midazolam) Liquid 0.5 mg/kg body weight 20 minutes before surgery: duration 2-3 hours
b)  Diazepam Tablet oral 2-10 mg 1 hour before surgery, duration of action 3 hours

**Intramuscular Medication for adults:**

a)  Diazepam 10 mg IM 15 minutes before surgery: Duration 1hour
b)  Midazolam (Dormicum, or versed) injection (0.5 to 2 mg may be given) 5 minutes before surgery : Duration 1 hour : This has more side effects and airway monitoring is required.

**Intravenous (IV) medication for adults:**

a)  Versed 2-4 mg : onset 1-2 minutes, duration 3-6 hours, dose dependent
b)  Fentinyl 50 mcg: onset 1-2 minutes, duration: 1-2 hours
C)  Propofol 50-75 mg: onset 30 seconds, duration 10 minutes: dose related

The above medications can be titrated to maintain maximum effect.

**Medication Preparation:**

**All medications come in single use packaging. Use the required dose and discard the unused medication.**

**Monitoring:**

a) Oxygen: the most important 2-4 L/ minute by nasal cannula

b) Pulse Oximeter monitor finger type on patient's index finger and monitor continuously.

c) Stethoscope with extension taped to chest to watch respirations

d) Blood pressure Cuff, on patient's arm and measure every 5 minutes

**Adverse Reactions of Anesthesia:**

1. If there is Bradycardia, according to ACL standards, is below 40 beats/minute give 0.2 mg Robinul IV or Atropine 0.2 mg IV and monitor

2. If there is Hypotension: Ephedrine 12.5 -25 mg IV

3. Emergency Hypertension: Labetolol 40 – 80 mg IV or Hydrolozine 10-40 mg IV or IM

4. Nausea: Zofran 4 mg IV or sublingual

**Resuscitation:**

1. Cardiac Arrest: Standard procedure for CPR

2. Ventilate patient, give vasopressor ephedrine 50 mg IV, CPR as necessary

3. Neosynephrine Flush for tachycardia with associated hypotension: Draw up Neosynephrine in 3 cc syringe, draw up 3 cc normal saline give IV. You may repeat this if necessary. This is very potent as it increases blood pressure and decreases heart rate.

**Acknowledgement: The part of the text was contributed by Steve Panter, who has extensive experience on ocular anesthesia, sedation and monitoring of ophthalmic surgery patients.**

# REFERENCES

1. Hay A, et al. Needle perforation of the globe during retrobulbar and peribulbar injection. Ophthalmology 1991;98: 1017-24.

2. Kimble JA, et al. Globe perforation from peribulbar injection. Arch Ophthalmol 1987;105: 749.

3. Shriver PA, et al. Effectiveness of retrobulbar and peribulbar anesthesia. J Cataract Ref Surg 1992;18: 162-65

4. Arora R, et al. Peribulbar anesthesia. J Cataract Ref Surg 1991; 17: 506-08.

5. Bloomberg L. Administration of periocular anesthesia. J Cataract Ref Surg 1986; 12: 677-79.

6. Davis DB. Posterior peribulbar anesthesia. J Cataract Ref Surg 1986;12: 182-84.

7. Gills JP, Cherchio M, Raanan MG. Unpreserved lidocaine to control discomfort during cataract surgery using topical anesthesia. J Cataract Refract Surg 1997;23: 545-50.

8. Koch PS. Anterior chamber irrigation with unpreserved lidocaine 1% for anesthesia during cataract surgery. J Cataract Refract Surg 1997;23: 551-54.

9. Fichman RA, Fine IH, Grabow HR. Clear-corneal Cataract Surgery and Topical Anesthesia Thorofare: Slack Inc. 1993.

10. Stevens JD. A new local anaesthesia technique for cataract extraction by one quadrant sub-Tenon's infiltration. Br J Ophthalmol 1992;76: 670.

11. Greenbaum S. Anesthesia in cataract surgery. In Greenbaum S (Ed): Ocular Anesthesia, Philadelphia: WB Saunders, 1997; 1-55.

12. Fukasaku H, Marron J A. Pin-point anesthesia—a new approach to local ocular anesthesia. J Cataract Refract Surg 1994;20:468.

## Chapter 7

# SICS MANUAL PHACO SURGERY

Learning Small Incision Cataract Surgery (SICS) and also ECCE (Extracapsular Cataract surgery) is essential for the surgeons in Developing countries and also for the cataract surgeons in the advanced countries.

There are several reasons for primarily choosing the SICS technique for cataract surgery. There are times when conversion to SICS becomes necessary while performing Phaco Surgery.

Although Phacoemulsification using the modern phaco machines and advanced materials is possible in all types of cataract cases by some surgeons, there are understandable limitations in performing surgery on hard nucleus when modern phaco machines and facilities are not available to the surgeon.

SICS OR ECCE MAY BE PREFERABLE IN THE FOLLOWING SITUATIONS:

1. Brunescent and Black Cataracts: These hard cataracts require excessive energy for phacoemulsification causing damage to cornea and the posterior capsule.
2. Hard Nucleus where attempted Chopping is not possible or there is an impending danger of corneal damage.
3. Morgagnian Cataract : These are Hypermature cataracts with weak zonules
4. Pseudo exfoliation Cataract with weak zonules
5. Cataract in eyes with shallow Anterior chamber
6. Cataract in Small Pupil with hard cataract cases
7. Mature Cataract with low Endothelial Cell Count

**SICS has the following advantages:**

Sutureless SICS has evolved as an effective alternative to phacoemulsification. Recent studies have shown that sutureless SICS is cost-effective and delivers comparable results in Cataract surgery.

## BENEFITS OF SUTURELESS SICS INCLUDE:

- Better and early wound stability than ECCE
- Less postoperative inflammation
- Avoidance of suture and suture-related complications (e.g., iris prolapse, suture infiltrate, bleeding)
- Fewer postoperative visits than ECCE.
- Reduced surgically induced astigmatism

Sutureless SICS and ECCE can be performed for most types of cataracts, in contrast to phacoemulsification in which case selection is important. In phacoemulsification, the duration of surgery and ultrasound power delivery for the emulsification of cataract varies with the nucleus density. On the other hand, with sutureless SICS, the time spent on nucleus delivery is largely uniform and does not vary from case to case. In cataracts with dense nuclei, with an incision size of 7 mm, the nucleus of any size and consistency can be easily delivered in most cases.

It is not possible to describe a generalized procedure for the SICS surgery because, the surgery depends on many variables and the surgeon must decide which procedure is best for which case. I shall therefore describe the different approaches adopted by different surgeons and it is up to the operating surgeon to decide which method is preferable for the particular case. In my opinion, the end result of the surgery is important. If the patient is happy with 6/6 vision after the post operative period, which procedure of lens delivery has been employed, whether sutures were used or which viscoelastic is used, becomes of secondary interest.

In order to learn Small Incision Cataract surgery, the surgeon has to understand the Mechanics of each step of the surgery.

### Steps of SICS (SMALL INCISION CATARACT SURGERY)

### A. Peritomy

The conjunctiva and the Tenon's layer are dissected separately or together. If necessary, very light cautery is used to stop bleeding from the superficial capillaries. If the surface is smooth, the scleral dissection becomes easier. The length of conjunctival dissection should be 8 to 10 mm. A fornix based flap is dissected but sometimes a limbus based flap may also be dissected.

**B. Superior Rectus Suture**: Many surgeons prefer to have a superior rectus bridle suture to stabilize the eye and to rotate the eye downwards, but this is not mandatory.

**C. Incision**:

Scleral Tunnel Incision is the preferred type of incision and has been described in the section of Incision. SICS can also be performed with Temporal Clear Corneal incision but it is better to use Scleral Tunnel incision.

Depending on the size of the Nucleus, a Scleral Frown incision is fashioned usually at the 12 o clock position. Other designs of external incision practiced are, Horizontal, V shaped, Horizontal incision with straight backward extensions. The entry may also be through the temporal side.

1.  A Scleral Tunnel about 6 mm to 7 mm in breadth and the center of the Frown is 1.5 mm from the limbus is dissected. A 300 Micron or Half scleral thickness scleral gutter is made vertically. Then a horizontal dissection is made in the sclera which proceeds forward up to the limbus. The dissection is performed with a Bevel up Crescent Blade.
2.  The incision is dissected forward into the cornea with the crescent knife for another 1.5 mm.
3.  The internal lip of the incision is dissected to 7.5 mm in breadth into the cornea. This dissection is important and has to be performed before entry is made into the anterior chamber.
4.  The Anterior chamber is entered with a Keratome by dipping the tip of the Keratome downwards. A corneal valve is made at this point. The relationship of the nucleus with the tunnel is most important. We must conceive the nucleus in the tunnel and its size, width and hardness while dissecting the tunnel. A too big tunnel will be redundant and a small tunnel will cause tissue damage and difficulty to deliver the nucleus.
5.  It is safer to fashion an adequate size incision and stitches given if required than to make a small size incision which is tight for nucleus delivery and will cause tissue damage, difficult or failed surgery.
6.  It is to be understood that the Tunnel is like the mouth of a Snake bigger inside and shorter on the outside.
7.  This type of incision is good enough for the delivery of most of the mature cataracts. The relationship of the width of the tunnel and the size of the nucleus is most important
8.  For very hyper mature cataract and Hard Nucleus the breadth of the incision may need to be wider up to 8 or 9 mm or so.

9.  The mechanics is to understand is in the construction of the Three Plane Corneo - Scleral valve incision, which will later be water tight upon closure at the end of the surgery. The internal lip of the corneal valve has to be intact for the incision to be water tight. When anterior chamber is reformed with BSS, the internal lip apposes to the outer lip to make the incision water tight. If the internal lip is damaged, ragged or otherwise malfunctions, the wound will not be water tight and sutures will be required. There are other factors responsible for making the wound water tight.

**D. Side Port:**

A standard side port incision is made about 2 clock hours away from the main incision into the Anterior Chamber with a 15 degree knife.

**E. Capsulotomy :**

1.  **CAPSULORHEXIS**: A capsulorhexis about 5.5 mm in diameter is performed. In order to perform the Rhexis, it is better to make a small entry through the main incision first. The anterior chamber is filled with viscoelastic. The Rhexis is started as a standard Phaco rhexis with a Cystitome and completed with a Rhexis forceps or the cystitome itself.

2.  **CAN OPENER CAPSULOTOMY**: SICS can also be performed through a Can Opener Capsulotomy or a D shaped open capsulotomy. If the Cataract is very Hypermature or Black Morgagnian cataract or Capsulorhexis is not possible for any reason, can opener capsulotomy may be performed. In this procedure a cystitome is fitted on a 3 cc syringe. The anterior chamber is filled with viscoelastic and small cuts are made in the anterior capsule 360 degrees and one cut is joined to the other and see that the capsulotomy is complete and there are no tags, at least 10 to 12 cuts are necessary to achieve a good capsulotomy. Unnecessary pull of the capsular tag will dislocate the whole bag. The perforated anterior capsule is then removed with a capsule holding forceps or a rhexis forceps. This creates a big opening for easy delivery of the Nucleus and the Posterior Capsule remains intact. The IOL has to be placed at the Sulcus.

**The mechanics in this step is to make the size of the Capsulorhexis or Capsulotomy according to the size of the Nucleus to be prolapsed into the anterior chamber.**

**F. Hydro procedures**: Hydrodissection produces a broad fluid wave that separates the epinucleus and the capsule. Nucleus disassembly then commences with hydrodelineation whereby a second internal fluid wave cleaves the epinucleus apart from the firmer endonucleus. There are three separate purposes served by hydrodissection: (1) endonucleus rotation, (2) epinucleus rotation, and (3) loosening of the cortex.

**Hydrodissection Goals**: Because the nucleus has to be prolapsed into the anterior chamber, nuclear rotation is integral to every SICS technique. Effective hydrodissection allows the nucleus to rotate with minimal stress upon the zonules. If the fluid wave passes along the inner capsular surface, it will accomplish the first two goals by separating the capsule from the epinucleus. As a result, both the epinucleus and endonucleus will rotate together — even following subsequent hydrodelineation.

**The mechanics of this step is to make the nucleus small enough by hydrodissection and hydrodelineation to be prolapsed easily through the opening in the anterior capsule created by capsulorhexis or capsulotomy.**

## G. PROLAPSE OF THE NUCLEUS INTO THE ANTERIOR CHAMBER:

This is one of the important steps; the nucleus must be prolapsed in to the anterior chamber safely in order to bring it outside the eye by expression. There are several ways to do this.

a) **Hydro Prolapse:** If you have performed a good Hydrodissection and hydrodelineation and if the cataract is grade 1 &2 the endonucleus will be small. Now take the hydro cannula filled with BSS and insert the cannula in between the epinucleus and the endonucleus. Inject gently some BSS and the nucleus will float up and will be prolapsed into the anterior chamber.

If the Nucleus is bigger than 5.5 MM, usually 6.5 mm or up, take a sinsky hook and tilt the nucleus by pressing on the side or at 3 O clock position. You will see the nucleus is tilting and the superior pole of the nucleus will come in front of the rhexis margin. Leave it there, next rotate the nucleus clockwise and you will see the nucleus is coming out of the bag into the anterior chamber and it will slide out of the bag into the A/C.

Many people take a cystitome and bury the tip of the cystitome into the nucleus to tilt it to bring one pole of the nucleus out of the bag to lie in front of the anterior capsule and then the procedure is the same, rotate the nucleus and it will come out of the bag to lie on the iris in the anterior chamber. Care is to be taken at this point so that, the cystitome does not penetrate the Capsulorhexis margin

If the nucleus is very big and cannot be prolapsed easily, make two small relaxing cuts in the upper part of the rhexis and tilt and prolapse the nucleus into the A/C in the same manner.

b) **Visco Prolapse** : This is described by Paul S. Koch and is a very clever but complex way to do it. After Capsulorhexis, using a curved cannula the tip of which is angled back 150 degrees which is called Corydon Cannula This cannula is introduced on a 3 cc syringe filled with BSS. The cannula is introduced just under the superior pole of the nucleus at 12 O clock position and a very gentle hydrodissection is performed carefully looking at the fluid wave. When the fluid wave reaches halfway through or 3 to 9 O'clock position, the hydrodissection is stopped. Now, a mechanical situation happens. The superior part of the nucleus is free but the inferior part of the Nucleus is still attached to the posterior capsule with cortex and therefore acts like a hinge. A little pressure on the nucleus allows the BSS to escape out. The point to understand at this situation is that, if the whole nucleus is hydro-dissected, it will lift up in the bag and cannot escape and any further pressure will cause the zonules to rip and the lens with the bag will dislocate. The Corydon Cannula is removed from the eye and now fitted on a 3 cc syringe filled with Viscoelastic. The Cannula is reinserted into the eye and positioned at the same plane of the nucleus at 12 O clock position. A small amount of Viscoelastic is injected in this position again looking carefully so that it reaches up to half position. At this point, with gentle pressure on the 6 o clock position, the nucleus will tilt against the pivot on the 6 O clock position and the superior pole of the nucleus will prolapse out of the bag.

Next move is to inject more viscoelastic or BSS under the nucleus to complete the hydrodissection at the same time sliding the nucleus out of the capsular bag by gentle rotation. Very gentle handling is the key to success to prolapse the nucleus in to the anterior chamber. Vigorous hydrodissection will create tear in the posterior capsule or whole nucleus with the bag to dislocate into the anterior chamber.

This procedure of Viscoexprerssion is very safe but need a lot of practice for the mechanics to work properly and has direct relationship to the size of the Rhexis and the size of the Nucleus. If the nucleus is too big, and cannot be prolapsed, a cut in the rhexis margin or a can opener capsulotomy is better.

If you have any doubt that the nucleus is hard and big, it is better to perform can opener capsulotomy rather than to risk the surgery. The nucleus may be prolapsed into the A/C in any of the mentioned procedures.

c) **Phaco divide and prolapse:** I have used this technique for nucleus delivery of hard cataracts many times. The initial incision is that of a phaco surgery where a 3.00 mm or 2.8 mm phaco incision with scleral tunnel is created. After routine Capsulorhexis and hydrodissection, a groove is made in the center of the nucleus. The nucleus is rotated and the groove is completed. The nucleus is divided into two halves using a spatula and the phaco tip or using spatula and a chopper. After the nucleus is divided into two halves, one half of the nucleus is held by phaco needle using high vacuum. The hemi nucleus is pulled into the anterior chamber and released. The first half of the nucleus can also be tumbled and rotated to be prolapsed into the anterior chamber manually. Second half of the nucleus is also brought into the anterior chamber using the same technique. This procedure has the advantage that the nucleus half is smaller and can be expressed through a relatively smaller incision and the result is that of a phaco surgery. The nucleus prolapse into the A/C is thus completed and the tunnel is now extended for nucleus expression.

## H. NUCLEUS EXPRESSION:

The next step is Expression of the nucleus out of the Anterior Chamber. The nucleus at this point is sitting on the Iris in the anterior chamber and is fully mobile.

The nucleus has to be brought out of the eye by some mechanism with minimum collateral damage. You have to understand that, there is a mismatch between the size of the wound and the size of the nucleus which has to come out. The nucleus is bigger than the width of the tunnel.

First step is to fill the anterior chamber with viscoelastic to coat the Endothelium properly so that the nucleus does not scratch the back of the cornea.

Next and most important step is to engage the edge of the nucleus into the mouth of the corneo scleral tunnel which is of adequate size to accommodate the nucleus.

The mechanics of nucleus expression is to increase the Pressure inside the anterior chamber so much that the nucleus is forced to come out of the anterior chamber, through the only natural passage it can move, the tunnel.

a) **Blumenthal Method**: Dr Blumenthal was a great thinker. I had met him several times in conferences, and his theory was to increase the pressure in the A/C by using an Anterior Chamber maintainer fitted through a stab incision at the lower part of the cornea and fluid enters the eye through the cannula by the force of gravity. While introducing the A/C maintainer, the irrigation must be on and the bevel must be down. Desmet's detachment is a complication of ACM. The pressure can be raised by increasing the bottle height. The internal hydrostatic pressure is maintained by the A/C maintainer. A Sheets Guide is next introduced behind the prolapsed nucleus in front of the Iris. This protects the iris from prolapsing into the wound. The fluid pressure engages the nucleus into the tunnel. At the same time a slight pull on the superior rectus bridle suture or depressing the outer lip of the scleral tunnel with toothed forceps tilts the nucleus out through the scleral tunnel. Pressure on the posterior lip of the tunnel with any instrument opens up the tunnel and delivers the nucleus.

b) **Viscoexprerssion:** In this process, Viscoelastic is injected into the anterior chamber through the side port and a slight traction is maintained with the Superior rectus suture. With the pressure of the viscoelastic thus injected and if the superior pole of the nucleus is engaged in the tunnel, it will wiggle out of the scleral wound with slight pressure on the outer lip of the scleral tunnel. If you press on the outer lip of the tunnel, it will open up and slide the nucleus out like passing the frog into a snake's mouth.

c) **Irrigating Vectis Method**: In this process, an Irrigating vectis is fitted on a 3 cc syringe filled with BSS. There are three ports of the vectis and it is to be tested for patency before introduction by pressing on the plunger. The Irrigating vectis can also be mounted on the Irrigating channel and the fluid pressure guided by raising the bottle height.

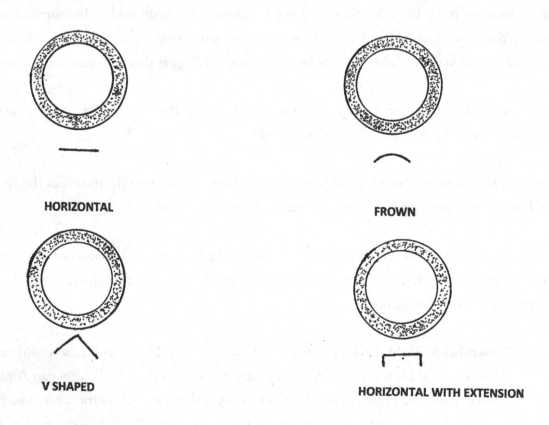

HORIZONTAL

FROWN

V SHAPED

HORIZONTAL WITH EXTENSION

Fig 11: (Types of Incisions in SICS)

Next, viscoelastic is injected below the Nucleus to push the posterior capsule and the anterior capsulorhexis margin down.

Introduce the Irrigating vectis under the nucleus carefully without touching the Iris or posterior capsule. Press on the plunger to push BSS into the anterior chamber and the nucleus will be pushed out through the scleral tunnel with a little pressure on the posterior lip of the scleral tunnel or pull of the Superior rectus suture.

d) **Fish Hook Method**: Some surgeons prefer to engage the nucleus with a specially prepared fish hook and remove the nucleus by pulling it out of the eye while exerting pressure holding the superior rectus suture with the other hand. The hook is made of a 30G Needle. The tip of the needle is bent 90 degrees which will be inserted into the nucleus. A second forward bend of the needle shaft is made for easy insertion of the hook into the substance of the nucleus. Viscoelastic is introduced into the A/C, the hook is introduced between the nucleus and the epinucleus with the needle tip pointing to the right side. The hook is then turned so that the needle tip engages the nucleus in the middle. The nucleus is then tilted and pulled out of the bag into the anterior chamber and pulled out of the anterior chamber through the tunnel without stopping. The epinucleus and cortex acts as a cushion and the nucleus is impaled is such a way that it do not rotate during extraction.

e) **Sandwich Technique**: In this technique, the nucleus is guided with two instruments, the vectis behind the nucleus and a spatula in front of the nucleus. Simultaneous pull of both the instruments will bring the nucleus out through the scleral tunnel. The second instrument also presses on the outer lip of the tunnel and facilitates the delivery of the nucleus. Here the important mechanics to mark is that, the sandwiched nucleus and the instruments act like a see-saw with fulcrum at the scleral lip. Very careful pull of both the instruments is required. The body of the see-saw has to be straight at the time of the pull to bring the nucleus out. Even slight tilting either way will damage the surrounding structures. Slight tilting up will damage the corneal endothelium, slight tilting down will damage the posterior capsule. Perfect balance is to be maintained while exerting pull of the instruments with the nucleus.

f) **The Snare method**: In Hypermature cataract with a big hard nucleus, the rhexis has to be big enough to prolapse it into the anterior chamber. It is not easy to do a 6.5 mm Rhexis safely, but when proficiency is gained, this can be performed in two steps, first a small 5 mm rhexis is made and nucleus is debulked by washing the liquid cortex, then a bigger rhexis is performed using the rhexis forceps and using Trypan Blue dye. The nucleus is prolapsed in the anterior chamber as described previously. The nucleus can then be bisected with a wire made Snare in to two or four pieces and the pieces delivered using Irrigating Vectis. This is an advanced technique of SICS and beginners should not try this method unless perfected under expert guidance. This procedure is reserved for big nucleus which is to be delivered through a small 4 or 5 mm scleral tunnel. The snare is made of a 28 G flexible stainless steel wire threaded through a 20 G disposable needle which is made blunt by cutting the tip off. The wire is sterilized by autoclaving. The loop snare thus prepared is introduced into the anterior chamber. The nucleus is introduced through the loop of the snare and the two ends of the snare are pulled to cut the nucleus into two halves. One half of the nucleus is then delivered through the scleral tunnel using irrigating vectis or by visco expression. The other half if the nucleus is treated in the same way. The snare may be used to create four pieces of the nucleus which are smaller and can easily be delivered through the tunnel.

g) **Phaco divide and expression:** This has already been described. The nucleus is divided into two halves using phaco machine after Capsulorhexis and hydrodissection. One half of the nucleus is then held by the phaco tip using high vacuum. This half is rotated out of the bag into the anterior chamber. The phaco tip is removed from the eye. The nucleus half is then oriented longitudinally in the anterior chamber and the incision is enlarged to a prefixed size of 5 to 5.5 mm. The superior tip of the hemi nucleus is engaged into the corneal valve of the tunnel. Viscoelastic like methyl cellulose is then injected to increase pressure in the anterior chamber which will push the piece out through the tunnel. The second half of the nucleus is still in the bag. There are two ways to tackle this half of the nucleus. Firstly, the eye is filled with viscoelastic and the remaining portion of the nucleus is slowly nudged with a sinsky hook to bring it out of the bag and then push it out of the Anterior Chamber with viscoelastic. Second method is to partially close the scleral incision with a 10/0 nylon suture and use the phaco probe with high vacuum setting to hold and to bring the piece out of the bag into the anterior chamber and leave it there. Next, the stitch is removed and the piece of the nucleus is expressed out with visco expression or irrigating vectis or any other method of nucleus removal. The advantage of this method is the smaller size of the incision required to deliver the nucleus and less astigmatism and more chance of making the incision sutureless.

**Mechanics:** Thus there are several methods for nucleus delivery, but one must understand the mechanics of it. There are four important mechanical considerations in this step.

**Firstly,** the internal wound must be bigger than the external wound in order to easily accommodate and engage the superior pole of the nucleus into the incision. Never insert any instrument like irrigating vectis and try to pull the nucleus out. If it does not engage into the wound, take a keratome and enlarge the internal side of the wound until it is big enough to accommodate the nucleus. You have to proportionately enlarge the outer side of the tunnel too to allow smooth nucleus delivery.

**Secondly**, you have to remember that you are delivering the nucleus through a tunnel. The superior pole of the nucleus has to come at the internal corneal side of the tunnel. There is no point in pushing the nucleus or injecting viscoelastic and inflating the A/C or the bag to burst it. Depress the outer lip of the tunnel, if the nucleus does not come easily to be engaged, use a second instrument to engage the superior pole of the nucleus into the corneal tunnel first. If you are using instrumental method like Irrigating Vectis, depress the outer lip of the tunnel for the nucleus to be engaged into the internal side of the incision and then introduce the instrument.

**Thirdly,** This is entirely a manual procedure and therefore, extreme care has to be taken to introduce, withdraw each instrument to minimize tissue damage. Desmet's detachment is a very important complication during instrumentation, Injury to Iris, Iris tear, corneal endothelial damage, Injury to the Capsular bag and even prolapse of the entire bag can happen. Therefore, every step has to be perfectly rehearsed and practiced, deliberate movements are carefully conducted under full visibility.

**Fourthly**, the construction of the tunnel has to be smooth, not ragged. A double tunnel or a ragged tunnel cannot give smooth delivery of the nucleus.

## I. CORTICAL ASPIRATION:

**Aspiration** of the cortex is the next step of SICS. This may be performed with a) Simco Cannula, mounted on an aspiration line and fitted with a 5 cc syringe. A smaller syringe do not produce enough vacuum, a larger one is difficult to manipulate. b) Automated Irrigation and Aspiration system used in Phaco Surgery.

Cortical cleaning in SICS or ECCE with Irrigation Aspiration system of Phaco machine need special preparation. As because the wound is big, it is not possible to create a closed atmosphere for vacuum to build up. In order to use an automated irrigation and aspiration system or any other mechanical system, the wound requires to be sutured first. The wound has to be partially closed keeping about 2.8 mm opening for the Irrigation and aspiration probe to go through. This means suturing the wound and the number of sutures will depend upon how big incision has been used to deliver the nucleus. After partially closing the incision, any automated I/A system can be used for cortical and epinucleus aspiration as described in Phaco surgery.

Cortical aspiration with simco cannula is a simple procedure, time tested and inexpensive.

First essential thing is to have a soft eyeball and a dilated pupil and clear visibility at all times. Adjust the microscope to see the cortical mater, posterior capsule, the rhexis margin at all times.

During the nucleus delivery, because of rubbing on the iris, the pupil may come down. Inject diluted Adrenaline into the anterior chamber and add half cc to the irrigating solution and this will dilate the pupil. Consent from the anesthetist is necessary for using Adrenaline into the anterior chamber.

Introduce the Simco cannula with the aspiration port facing you (upwards), start the irrigation, you will see a lots of cortical mater floating in the anterior chamber. Aspirate one strand of the cortex strip it towards the center and under direct visibility, increase the vacuum by pulling on the plunger of the syringe and aspirate the whole of it.

I usually hold the cannula with the right hand in between my index and thumb and balance with middle finger. I hold the syringe with the left hand and the plunger in between the thumb and the index fingers of my left palm.

In Hypermature cataracts it is easy to aspirate the cortex because very little cortex is left behind and is milky and soft; gentle irrigation brings out most of it for aspiration. In mature and immature cataracts where a lot of cortical mater is left behind, patience is required. Surgical success depends upon full cortical removal. Left over cortical mater gives rise to inflammation in the postoperative period and posterior capsule opacity.

First thing is to insert the cannula with irrigation fully on.

1. Move your cannula to the 6 O'clock position near the edge of the pupil. Gently aspirate some cortical matter in the cannula. Now stop aspirating but keep the suction on. Pull the cortex towards the centre. A triangular cortex will be stripped. The base of the triangle is towards the iris and apex towards the centre. Now suck the loosened cortex in the cannula. Don't suck until it is free.

2. Now move the tip of your cannula to seven O'clock position. Repeat the same process of stripping. You will find a clear area. This structure less clear area is floored by posterior capsule.

3. Sometimes you will find that the cortex is adherent & it does not enter the port even on good sucking. In these cases do not aspirate. Just keep irrigating, in the bag, behind the iris. If you have patience, a chunk of the cortical matter will be loose and float freely. Thereafter it becomes easy to strip and aspirate the cortex.

4. Move your cannula to 4 O'clock position. Suck a bit of cortical flap & pull again. Another triangular cortical matter will be stripped. Now you will have a bigger triangle floored by the posterior capsule.

5. Do not go toward the posterior capsule. You have no business there. Going near it is dangerous at this stage.

6. It is also dangerous to try to strip the cortex from the centre.

7. Always start stripping from the pupillary margin and under the Capsulorhexis margin with full visibility.

8. Irrigate behind the iris. When cortex becomes loose aspirates it & strip it.

9. Every time you are aspirating, check that the port is upward, facing you, or facing sideways. Never suck when the port is facing the posterior capsule.

10. When the lower part has been cleared, come to 3 O'clock position. Aspirate the cortex & strip it as before. A little side to side movement while you are holding the cortical tag helps to free a big chunk of cortical matter.

11. While stripping the cortex, remember that, if you suck too hard, you will ingest a cortical fragment. The rest of it will break & go behind the iris inside the bag & it is difficult to pick it up again at these positions, therefore strip it before aspirating.

12. Go to 9 O'clock position & repeat the procedure. If a big chunk is about to come, a little rotary, side to-side movement will help to free it up.

13. The top position is difficult to clear. Go to 12 O'clock position and try to strip downwards. If there is a big chunk of cortical matter at 12 O'clock position, it is easy to strip it. However if there is very small amount of cortical matter deep behind the iris, it is difficult to get hold of it & difficult to aspirate it.

14. In this situation, take a curved single way irrigating cannula & irrigate at the 12 O'clock position under the upper part of capsular bag. This will loosen any cortex left deep inside the bag at 12 O clock position. Next, take a two-way simco cannula and aspirate by stripping the cortical mater as before. If you are using a curved simco cannula it may be easier. If there is a very small amount of cortical matter deep behind the iris in the upper

part of the bag, it may not be necessary to clean it. But the posterior capsule must be clean and clear.

The Mechanics of Aspiration of Cortex is simple but important. The residual cortex must be floated and striped to the center for aspiration. The Posterior capsule must be cared for and always kept in view so that it is not injured. You will need to bring the cannula out of the A/C several times to empty the syringe when it is full. Always try to leave a formed A/C or inject viscoelastics to reform the A/C before further manipulations. Protection of the cornea and the Posterior capsule is most important at this stage.

**J. Implantation of the IOL**: Next step is the implantation of the intraocular lens. It is simple in SICS and ECCE. If there is an intact Rhexis, Foldable Lens can be implanted. The modern Acrylic Foldable Lenses are far superior in terms of biocompatibility and results in less postoperative inflammation than the PMMA lenses. However, a good quality PMMA Lens will also give good and comparable post operative result.

Reform the Anterior chamber and the bag with Viscoelastics. Just hold the IOL with a lens holding forceps at the Optic and insert the IOL if the incision is bigger than the optic size of the IOL. Most IOL s are 5.5 to 6mm in diameter and this can be directly implanted if the incision size is 6.5 mm. or more. In case, the incision size is less than 5.5 mm, the Foldable IOL can be implanted with the injector. If using a rigid PMMA IOL, the incision needs to be enlarged to 6mm in size.

**The Correct Plane**

If the bag is intact, the lens must be placed in the bag

In case of sulcus fixation or when can -opener capsulotomy has been done, the ciliary sulcus is the anatomical entity where you are going to place the loops of the lens. This is between the posterior iris root and the ciliary body. Subsequently fibrosis fixes the lens permanently. You will find it is surprisingly easy to implant the lens at the correct position provided that the conditions for implantation are ideal.

Follow the following steps for insertion of a rigid PMMA IOL:

1. Inject enough viscoelastic in the anterior chamber. The chamber should be fully formed.

2. Make sure that the pupil is dilated and cornea is clear. You can see the posterior capsule against a red reflex. If the pupil is not dilated, inject diluted cardiac Adrenaline to dilate the pupil. Be careful with cardiac or hypertensive patients.

3. Ask the nurse to open the packet of the implant & wash the implant with Ringers or BSS.

4. Pick it up with a McPherson forceps

5. Grasp the optic at the optic & upper haptic junction with a lens holding forceps or an angled McPherson forceps with your right hand.

6. Tell the nurse to put a blob of viscous substance on the lens & haptic.

7. Lift the edge of anterior scleral lip with your left hand with a plane forceps. As soon as you have placed the inferior loop at the upper part of anterior chamber release the scleral flap.

8. The correct way to hold the lens with the McPherson forceps is between the thumb, index & middle fingers with your hand in pronation.

9. Insert the inferior loop at an angle of 10 degrees downwards. Go through the anterior chamber at the iris plane.

10. The angle of the McPherson forceps should be at your right, and hand in pronation. The inferior loop will go smoothly behind the iris at 6 O'clock position in the bag or the sulcus as the case may be. Now release your grip at the optic.

11. Now two things may happen. One, the lens may remain at the place you have just placed it. This is ideal and you proceed as described below. The lens may slide out if there is back pressure because the wound is not a closed wound like we find in Phacosurgery,

12. If the inferior haptic is in position behind the iris & you have released the lens grip at the optic, don't push it any further. If you push any further, it is going to injure the Zonule or the posterior capsule and you will observe a "setting sun"!

13. Now hold the McPherson forceps with your right hand in supination and the angle of the forceps to the left.

14. With the closed tips of the forceps nudge the superior pole of the optic gently and slowly. Gradually nudge the optic completely in the anterior chamber. At this position you will have the superior haptic just outside the wound. Rest of the lens will be within the anterior chamber, either in the bag or the sulcus as the case may be.

15. The next step is to insert the upper loop. You can do it in two ways with a semi closed chamber; you can insert a lens dialer into the dialing hole of the optic if there is one or the optic haptic junction if there is no hole & dial clockwise. Rotate the lens slowly

without exerting downward pressure keep on rotating, keep on. The lens will rotate & the upper loop will automatically go in the bag. Rotate further to bring the lens loops in the horizontal position.

The second option is to grasp the tip of the upper loop with the tip of McPherson's forceps. Bend the loop and take the forceps to 3 O'clock position slightly rotate the tip of the forceps to place the end of the haptic just behind the iris in the bag and release it. The loop will spring up inside the bag or the sulcus.

16. The key point is, do not push the optic or the body of the lens below the horizontal. If the lens is placed in the sulcus and the optic or the haptic is pushed downward, there will be zonular dehiscence & vitreous prolapse with the attending problems.

17. Dialing is not essential but better. Insert the dialer & dial 20 degrees and Repeat this until you are satisfied with the position of the IOL.

18. To perform a "tap test" gently Introduce the dialer into a hole or body of the optic & gently push the lens down. The lens will spring back.

19. If you have difficulty to insert the upper loop in these methods, especially if there is a back pressure, and every time you try to push the lens, it comes out of the bag or sulcus due to back pressure, don't despair. You have other options to insert the upper loop and position the lens properly. This happens because the incision in SICS is big and the chamber is not closed as in Phaco surgery. Reform the anterior chamber with viscoelastic; hold the upper loop at its tip with McPherson forceps with your right hand. Take an iris retractor in your left hand. Gently retract the iris and place the upper loop behind the iris into the upper edge of the capsulorhexis and release the loop. It will spring up at the proper position. Release the iris from the retractor. Reposit the iris with an iris repositor. Fill the Anterior Chamber with viscoelastic and dial the lens into the bag.

The loops will go in position in the bag. Remember that if you have introduced the loop in this manner, dialing is a must after reforming the anterior chamber with viscoelastics. This is the worst of all the processes of lens insertion & there is danger of disinsertion of iris and many other complications. However you may have to take this last option if all other techniques to implant the IOL have failed.

20. Insertion of a foldable acrylic IOL with an injector through a 5.5 mm incision is the same as in Phacoemulsification. It is easier to implant foldable IOL if the incision is smaller and the capsular bag is intact. With a 5 mm or a 5 mm incision, the tip of the injector is inserted into the anterior camber and brought to the center of the chamber. The lens is pushed out of the injector slowly and the lower loop is introduced in the bag. The lens is then delivered in the anterior chamber and dialed slowly into the bag.

## K. Closure of the wound

The final step in SICS is closure of the wound. Aspirate as much viscoelastic as possible using simco cannula or an automated irrigation aspiration system from the anterior chamber. Next refill the anterior chamber with BSS through the side port. Refilling the anterior chamber will exert pressure on the corneal lip of the incision and the incision will self close. Test this with cotton swab or sponge at the external surface of the wound and you will find that there is no leak of BSS from the wound.

If still there is leakage of BSS from the external part of the wound, hydrate the wound with BSS. A blunt tip cannula is taken fitted on a syringe filled with BSS. The cannula is pressed at the side of the wound and corneal side of the wound is hydrated. The hydrated cornea swells up and the wound closes and leaking is stopped. Check this with a sponge.

If the wound is still leaking and you cannot close in spite of all your efforts, put one stitch with 10/0 Nylon at 12 o clock position and test again. If not sealed yet, put one suture on each side of the first suture and test for leak until this is water tight. Bury the knot of the suture into the wound by rotating the suture with McPherson's forceps. This does not irritate or cause any harm to the patient.

Remember, never be afraid to put stitches to close the wound properly, you can remove the stitch four to six weeks after surgery and the surgery will be suture less.

But if you leave a leaking wound, Shallow Anterior chamber, soft eyeball and all the other complications will follow. It is also difficult to close the wound afterwards because the tissue becomes fragile.

Don't be shy or afraid to put one or two sutures at the end of surgery should you detect a leaking wound. I have done this on many occasions: simply explain to the patient that "The cataract was very hard and I had to insert few safety sutures for the safety of your eye and vision, which can be removed after 6 weeks, there were no operative complications". I describe these stitches as safety sutures so that on post operative visits if the patient goes to another doctor, the patient knows that there are stitches to close the wound and do not get a disappointment. No patient ever complained to me about this. But it is very hard to explain the cause of a leaking wound and the necessity of putting sutures the day after surgery.

**EXTRACAPSULAR CATARACT EXTRACTION AND PC IOL IMPLANTATION (ECCE with PC IOL) :** Although this is obsolete procedure now and many surgeons will not be acquainted with the procedure any longer, I think it is necessary for an expert surgeon to learn about the procedure. In certain situation, this procedure may be a life saver for the surgeon. ECCE may be performed in the following situations: 1) if during phaco surgery, conversion becomes necessary due to any reason, ECCE can safely be performed. 2) If the cataract is so much Hypermature that it is black and hard with a big nucleus SICS may not be safe and in this situation, ECCE can be performed. Basically, whenever Phaco or SICS cannot be performed or is unsafe, ECCE can easily be performed. I shall give a brief outline of the procedure which is not much different from SICS. The surgery is performed under regional local anesthesia.

## STEPS OF ECCE

1) Firstly a small direct entry incision is given at the corneo scleral limbus to enter the anterior chamber.2) Viscoelastic is introduced to fill the anterior chamber.3) A can opener capsulotomy is performed preferably using dye. The tags of the anterior capsule are removed with a McPherson forceps. 4) The wound is enlarged using Right and Left corneal enlarging scissors (if this is not available, an universal enlarging scissors may be used) taking care so that enlarging incision is placed along the limbus. 5) Hydrodissection is performed to make the nucleus mobile. 6) Viscoelastic is again introduced to fill the anterior chamber.7) The nucleus is expressed using pressure at 6 o clock position with counter pressure at the wound margin.8) Irrigation and aspiration is performed using Simco Cannula to remove the residual cortical mater. It is to be remembered that, the wound is a big 10 to 11 mm in diameter and the A/C is open all the time and care is to be taken during this step not to injure the cornea or posterior capsule.9) A PMMA intraocular lens is implanted in the sulcus as because the bag is open. The upper loop is dialed to bring it to horizontal position. 10) The pupil should be constricted using intracameral preservative free Myochol or Pilocarpine.11) The wound is closed with 10/0 Nylon interrupted sutures.12) The A/C is reformed with BSS. 12) The knots of the suture ends are buried into the corneal stroma with curved McPhersons forceps. 13) Antibiotics drops and Pad and Shield are applied.

## References

1.  Gogate P M, Deshpande M, Wormald R P. Is manual small incision cataract surgery affordable in the developing countries? A cost comparison with extracapsular cataract extraction. Br J Ophthalmol. 2003;87:843–846. [PMC free article] [PubMed]

2. Hennig A, Kumar J, Yorston D, Foster A. Sutureless cataract surgery with nucleus extraction: Outcome of a prospective study in Nepal. Br J Ophthalmol. 2003;87(3):266–270. [PMC free article] [PubMed]

3. Natchiar G. Madurai, India: Aravind Publications; 2000. Manual Small Incision Cataract Surgery.

4. Ruit S, Poudyal G, Gurung R, Tabin G, Moran D, Brian G. An innovation in developing world cataract surgery: sutureless extracapsular cataract extraction with intraocular lens implantation. Clin Experiment Ophthalmol. 2000;28:274–279. [PubMed]

5. Thomas R, Kuriakose T, George R. Towards achieving small-incision cataract surgery 99.8% of the time. Indian J Ophthalmol. 2000;48:145–151. [PubMed]

6. Blumenthal M. Manual ECCE, the present state of the art. Klin Monat Augenheilkd. 1994;205:266–270.

7. Kansas P. Phacofracture. In: Rozakis GW, Anis AY, et al., editors. Cataract Surgery: Alternative Small Incision Techniques. Thorofare (N.J): Slack Inc; 1990. pp. p. 45–70.

8. Fry LL. The Phacosandwich Technique. In: Rozakis GW, Anis AY, et al., editors. Cataract Surgery: Alternative Small Incision Techniques. Thorofare (N.J): Slack Inc; 1990. pp. p.71–110.

9. Hennig A, Kumar J, Singh AK, Singh S, Gurung R, Foster A. World Sight Day and cataract blindness. Br J Ophthalmol. 2002;86:830–831. [PMC free article] [PubMed]

10. Prajna NV, Chandrakanth KS, Kim R, Narendran V, Selvakumar S, Rohini G, et al. The Madurai intraocular lens study II: clinical outcomes. Am J Ophthalmol. 1998;125:14–25. [PubMed]

11. Gogate P M, Deshpande M, Wormald R P, Deshpande R D, Kulkarni S R. Extracapsular cataract surgery compared with manual small incision cataract surgery in community eye care setting in Western India: a randomized controlled trial. Br J Ophthalmol. 2003;87:667–672. [PMC free article] [PubMed]

12. Keener GT. The nucleus division technique for small incision cataract extraction. In: Rozakis GW, Anis AY, et al., editors. Cataract Surgery: Alternative Small Incision Techniques. Thorofare (N.J): Slack Inc; 1990. pp. p.163–195.

13. S.M.Munirul Huq aand Karl Holzinger, Essentials of Cataract and Lens Implant Surgery : Jesmine Publications, Dhaka Bangladesh

# Chapter 8
# STEPS OF PHACO SURGERY

Phacoemulsification surgery requires few instruments and equipments and specific techniques which are to be mastered by repeated practice. The more understanding about the techniques is gained, the surgeon becomes more proficient. Every step of the surgery has to be exact because problem in one step makes the next step more difficult. The steps of the surgical procedure can be summarized as follows:

**STEPS BEFORE THE SURGERY STARTS:**

1. On arrival, take consent for surgery signed by the patient or next of keen
2. Dilate the patient with Tropicamide 1% and phenylephrine 10 % eye drops add NSID like indomethacin or similar eye drops and a broad spectrum antibiotics eye drops one hour before the surgery.
3. Examine the patient and decide on the type of anesthesia required, Topical or Regional.
4. In the Operation Room, check how easily the patient can lie flat on the table, if there is discomfort, find out what it is and make the patient absolutely comfortable, if necessary raise the head of the patient.
5. Examine the nucleus under the microscope and assess the hardness of the cataract and the type of opacity and decide for the last time about anesthesia and install the appropriate anesthesia required.
6. Check Blood Pressure, Vital Sign Monitors, Oxygen tube, and sterile sheet to cover the patient.
7. Put few drops of Betadine and topical anesthetic, clean the orbital area, drape the patient and insert a wire eye speculum.
8. The surgeon in now seated comfortably and microscope adjusted and Foot Plate of the phaco machine and Foot plate of the Microscope are placed in appropriate positions.
9. Wash the Betadine by irrigating with BSS and if performing clear corneal tunnel incision, mark the appropriate site for the entry incision.

**Eight STEPS OF PHACO SURGERY: As described by Dr. Matti Vazeen:**

1. **Incision**
2. **Introduction of Viscoelastic**
3. **Rhexis**
4. **Hydrodissection and Rotation of Nucleus**
5. **Phacoemulsification and removal of Nucleus**
6. **Irrigation and Aspiration of Cortex**
7. **Introduction of IOL**
8. **Wound Hydration and closure**

**Memorize these 8 steps of Phaco surgery well so that each step comes naturally one after the other.**

## ELABORATION OF THE STEPS:

1. For corneal tunnel incision make a groove parallel to the limbus take a 2.8 or a 3.1 mm sharp keratome and advance the keratome into the corneal stroma for about 2.5 mm parallel to the iris and then the tip of the keratome is directed downwards to enter the eye. A small amount of aqueous will escape to confirm that the anterior chamber is entered while care is taken not to injure the Iris or the Lens.

2. The eye is filled with viscoelastics and the Paracentesis tract is made with a 15 degree knife taken in the non dominant hand and the anterior chamber is entered near the limbus, parallel to the iris plane. The purpose of the side port is to introduce the second instrument and viscoelastics. Fill the eye with Viscoelastic again.

3. Inject viscoelastic to make the eye ball firm and introduce the Cystitome or Utrata Forceps to start Capsulorhexis and complete a 5 mm or a 5.5 mm round CCC. If viscoelastic escapes from the A/C, reform the anterior chamber by injecting more viscoelastic. Avoid posterior vitreous pressure rise which will force the rhexis to redialize, grasp every two clock hours and move the forceps to create a round and intact rhexis edge.

4. Take a 2.5 cc syringe filled with BSS and attach a hydrodissection cannula. Take the syringe in the dominant hand in pronation and press the outer lip of the main incision to egress some viscoelastic. The eye ball should be soft at this point and insert the cannula to create a hydrodissection. If fluid wave is seen to propagate beneath the nucleus, let it pass smoothly and then press slightly on the nucleus with the elbow of the cannula to allow some BSS to escape from the capsular bag. Further hydrodelineation and other hydro

procedures are optional procedures and performed according to the need and preference of the surgeon. See whether the nucleus rotates easily or not.

5. Hold the phaco handpiece with your Dominant hand just like holding pen to write, keep all the weight of the hand piece on your pronated wrist. Insert the phaco tip inside the anterior chamber with bevel up. Depress the Foot paddle to position 1 and the A/C will fill up with irrigating BSS. Depress the foot Plate to Position2 and bring the phaco tip to the surface of the nucleus to touch, don't press on the nucleus or push it. Firmly keeping the touch and tip directed downwards press the foot paddles to position 2.5 and further to position III(3). A shoo choo sound will be heard and you have started the Phaco surgery. By firmly holding the phaco handpiece continue to perform phaco in foot position 3 and a groove will be created from the center of the nucleus to 6 O clock positions. Next, rotate the nucleus and complete the trench from 12 O clock to 6 O clock position. Proceed to nucleus removal in one of the methods described. The Techniques for nucleus removal are, Spring Surgery or Chip and Flip Technique, Trench or Crater Divide and Conquer technique, Four Quadrant Divide and Conquer Technique, Stop and Chop Technique, Stop Chop and Stuff technique, Nonstop Phaco Chop Technique. Chose the technique that you think is best for the particular patient. Note that the texture of the Nucleus becomes smooth when the right depth is reached and the red glow is visible.

6. After the Nucleus is removed, the Epinucleus and the cortical mater need removal. Change parameters of the phaco machine and remove the Epinucleus and in most cases both Epinucleus and cortex will be removed together. We need very little intermittent phaco power but high vacuum and flow. Next you will need to remove the residual cortical mater by the I/A handpiece, switch the phaco handpiece to I/A handpiece change the phaco parameters to I/A mode and do the I/A carefully, remember, most or the accidents of posterior capsule rupture happens at this step. If you are not sure, and practicing, do Irrigation and aspiration with SIMCO cannula for the first few cases. Watch for: Stress lines in the posterior capsule. This indicates that the posterior capsule is engaged in the handpiece, do not move your handpiece, stop aspiration and go into irrigation or activate reflux of the machine. Hopefully the capsule will be released without break. Be careful while removing all the cortical mater from the sub incisional area.

7. Fill the eye with viscoelastic so that the bag is fully formed and the posterior capsule is pushed backwards. Take the Foldable IOL in the injector; the acrylic lens will already be in the injector by the nurse. You may widen the wound a small amount on one or both sides of the wound for easy entry of the tip of the injector through the wound. Place tip of inserter with bevel down into the wound. Use a gentle rotating motion to advance the tip into the anterior chamber. The plunger may need rotation or push depending

upon manufacturer Company specification to deliver the IOL. Continue to push until the entire lens passes through the tip. The injector is elevated so that the tip is oriented slightly posteriorly and the leading haptic and leading edge of lens will be in capsular bag. Gently remove the inserter, and the lens will begin to unfold. Engage the trailing haptic with a Sinsky hook or a lens manipulator. Gently place the elbow of the haptic under the anterior capsule using the sinsky hook. As the lens unfolds, the whole lens will be in the capsular bag. In order to remove the viscoelastics from the anterior chamber, take the I/A handpiece once again and introduce the I/A tip into the anterior chamber and do standard irrigation and aspiration until all the viscoelastics have been removed.

8. Place a 3cc syringe with irrigating cannula through the side port. Irrigate BSS to reform the anterior chamber. The globe should be firm. Remove the cannula and check the wound for leaks. Hydrate the wound to make it water tight. Place a few drops of antibiotics in the conjunctival sac, remove the speculum, remove the drape and the patient may be transported to the waiting area. Pad and shield is optional.

**It is easy to practice these 8 steps repeatedly until full proficiency is gained**.

Goat's eyes, Pig Eyes, Artificial Acrylic Practice eyes or Cadaver eyes may be used to practice. Fresh Cadaver eye is difficult to get for this purpose in our country but goat's eyes or Pig's eyes are easy to get and one can practice these 8 steps easily on these eyes. Preparation of these enucleated practice eyes is important. As because these practice eyes do not have the natural muscle tone they are soft and difficult to work on. They need to be mounted on a special stand or a stand prepared indigenously which can squeeze and give the necessary firmness to the structure to work on. They may be held firmly in a container by an assistant to give it a firm to touch feeling to practice the steps. It is also important to remember that, these eyes has a soft lens and only spring surgery or chip and flip procedure can be performed with these eyes. However, Incision, Rhexis, Hydro procedures, and starting to the make the groove can be practiced also Irrigation and Aspiration and striping of the cortex including implantation of an IOL can be adequately practiced. At least 50 practice surgeries on these eyes should be performed before starting an actual surgery on live patients. This is an arbitrary number for guidance only. The protocol may be different in different centers.

While performing surgery in the first 50 live cases, an experienced guide surgeon should be assisting to ensure safety. It is not enough only to assist a surgeon, it is important to practice the steps of the surgery which becomes next to habit and also see how the experienced surgeon manages the difficult situations. But it is most important that the learner surgeon does at least

50 practice surgery cases with practice eyes under supervision to learn the steps of the surgery and learn the control the machine. Then perform 50 live surgeries under supervision while the trainer surgeon actually assists the trainee to perform the surgery. In order to become proficient and to perform the surgery safely, I feel this protocol is necessary. This book and other books will explain the sequence of the steps and the procedure to perform them but the surgeon must perform the steps with actual machine and under actual situations and guidance. It is not difficult to learn Phacosurgery, but needs strong commitment and repeated practice to perform the steps accurately and safely to deliver good results.

## IMPORTANT NOTES FOR BEGINNER SURGEONS:

While converting from ECCE or SICS to phaco surgery, the surgeon will first feel a sudden increase in the speed of the surgery. This is like driving a car which suddenly takes up a speed from 10 mph to 60 mph on a racing track. Therefore the surgeon must stay focused and should continually be aware of what instrument is being used and how much that instrument can be moved inside the eye ball without causing collateral damage to other structures at every step of the surgery. **The second most important point for a beginner surgeon is to remember that, each step of phaco surgery is built upon the previous step**. If one step does not go as planned, the rest of all the steps become difficult. What we mean by that is, for example, if the incision that is supposed to be 2.8 mm and is made 3.8 mm, this just one mm difference in incision size will cause the wound to be loose fitted to the phaco probe with sleeves and BSS will leak from the sides of the wound resulting in instability of the anterior chamber depth. This may lead to difficulty in removing the nuclear fragments with a potential danger for a break in the capsule or zonular tear. A properly constructed incision leads to easier removal of the nucleus and a stable chamber. This concept is simple but overlooked frequently. The point to emphasize here is, at each step the beginner surgeon should pause, memorize the step and understand what it means to be done properly.

## EACH STEP IS BUILT UPON THE PREVIOUS STEP AND FOLLOWS THE STEPS SEQUENTIALLY.

Do not past go to the next step until the previous step has been completed to your satisfaction and perfection. Patience at every step of the surgery is important for the beginner. If hydrodissection is not done properly, the nucleus will not rotate and removal of the nucleus and cortex will be difficult. Trying to rotate the nucleus forcibly will invariably create problems. Eye surgeons are not robots and we perform surgery on a very complex human structure, the eye with the help of a very advanced computerized machine. Therefore, complications can happen. The key to a great outcome is recognition of the problem as it happens and the surgeon performs the necessary adjustments to compensate for the problem in the steps that follow the complication.

If for example, the incision is larger than planned, adjustments can be done by slowing the surgical speed down, raise the bottle height to increase flow rate to compensate for the leakage of fluid, do a good hydrodissection to ensure rotation of the nucleus, use plenty of viscoelastics and try to maintain a deep anterior chamber all the time. The vacuum should be adjusted so that there is minimum fluctuation of the anterior chamber and the surgery can be completed with no further complications. The cataract surgery can be broken down to millimeter steps. It becomes lot more easy if one tries to memorize the small millimeter steps, and practice these steps repeatedly to perfection before going to the next step. When these millimeter steps are performed accurately and added together, this gives excellent results. When performed with precision, Cataract surgery can become poetry in motion. When performed improperly this may become an unbelievable struggle with unpredictable outcome.

# Chapter 9
# PHACO INCISIONS

When Intracapsular Cataract extraction (ICCE) and Extracapsular Cataract Extraction ECCE) with IOL implantation was the choice of surgery in 1970 and 1980s, a large incision 10 to 12 mm at the Corneo-scleral Limbus was the incision of choice to enter the anterior chamber. This large incision was necessary to extract the Nucleus or the whole lens and to insert the PMMA Intraocular lens and the wound used to be secured with 10/O Nylon interrupted or continuous sutures. Direct entry incision with a blade or diamond knife were used which had no valve effect and required sutures for wound apposition and healing. The wound had to be enlarged with Right and Left cutting corneal scissors to the desired size. The post operative result used to be good but with a large post operative Astigmatism with the rule. Six weeks after the surgery, the stitches could be removed which would reduce the Astigmatism but still some residual astigmatism would be left behind.

After Phaco surgery was popularized in early 1990 s, the incision size was reduced to 3.5 mm and this reduced the Astigmatism but it was not astigmatically neutral. The incision to enter the eye today is sutureless self sealing, three step incision with a corneal valve. The entry incision may be planned as Scleral Tunnel or a Clear Corneal Tunnel incision depending upon the type of surgery being performed.

**Sutureless self sealing Incisions** for Cataract surgery is essentially a Three Step Incision and can be planned as:

1. Scleral Tunnel Incision
2. Clear corneal Tunnel Incision based on Limbus.
3. Clear corneal valve incision in front of limbus.

Both the corneal tunnel or scleral tunnel incision has advantages and disadvantages and it is recommended that the beginner surgeon learns the physics and constructions of both the types of incisions. The surgeon can then decide which type of entry will be good for a particular patient.

In some cases, a choice of incision may also help to reduce the pre-existing Astigmatism and toricity of the cornea. Some surgeons also use corneal relaxing incisions to treat pre-existing corneal astigmatism.

**Scleral Tunnel Incision:**

The classical Scleral Tunnel incision is a three –step incision shaped like a "Z". The three steps are: 1) The Vertical Gutter at the external site at the sclera, 2) Horizontal dissection extending into the cornea, 3) Angled entry to the anterior chamber with formation of a corneal valve.

**Fixation of the eye:**

For Scleral Tunnel, incision has to be placed at 12 O'clock position and therefore a Superior Rectus Bridle Suture is required to rotate the eye downwards.

A Parabulbar Injection local anesthesia or, regional local anesthesia is preferred over Topical Anesthesia in this type of incision and the reason being, the surgery tends to take longer to complete and conjunctival incision is painful.

**Conjunctival incision:**

A fornix based conjunctival flap is dissected with Tenon's capsule and blunt dissection is performed into the sub-tennon's space with blunt scissors. Mild cautery is applied to the superficial bleeding capillaries using a bipolar cautery.

**Site of the External Incision**

The site of the external Scleral incision should be 1.5 mm posterior to the Limbus, measured by a caliper and 2.8 to 3.5 mm in length.

**Type of the Scleral Incision:**

The scleral incision may be: 1) In the form of a straight line 2) Shaped like a Frown 3) Parallel to the Limbus 4) Horizontal with backward extension. The breadth of the incision depends upon the Optic size of the IOL, usually 2.8 mm to 5.5 mm.

**Thickness of the Tunnel:**

The tunnel incision should be 300 micron deep, or half sclera thickness. This can be done with a prefixed knife or by normal Razor blade fragment on a fragment holder. Exact depth has to be practiced beforehand. Too thin a tunnel may cause button hole of roof, too deep tunnel may cause inadvertent entry to the anterior chamber.

**Length of Tunnel:**

The corneo-scleral tunnel length is commonly done 2.5 mm well advanced in the cornea. This can be measured with caliper or prefixed keratome may be used

**Technique of making the Incision**

1) Firstly, conjunctiva is reflected and light cautery applied. Caliper is used to mark the length of the incision, a preset 300 Micron blade is used to make the initial incision into the sclera, the center of the frown is 1.5 mm behind the Limbus and the sides of the frown is more posterior. If a straight line incision is made, the whole incision is 1.5 mm behind the Limbus.

2) Next a Crescent Knife is taken and scleral dissection is made keeping the knife at the correct depth and pushed forward and sideways with a zigzag motion so that the depth of the incision is the same throughout the tunnel. With experience one can judge the depth of the tunnel by seeing the crescent blade through the roof of the tunnel. The tunnel is carried forward for 2.5 to 3 mm, which means 1 mm to 1.5 mm into the clear cornea and the Crescent knife is withdrawn.

3) The suitable size Keratome is next taken and passed smoothly through the tunnel. At this point care should be taken so that the Keratome do not proceed in a wrong direction to create a ragged incision or another track. When the tip of the Keratome reaches the end of the tunnel, it is advanced into the clear cornea and at the appropriate intended point of entry is reached., The tip of the keratome is then dipped posteriorly and advanced slowly until it appears into the anterior chamber, the direction of the blade is again turned horizontal and the entry is completed.

   Sudden push at this stage is dangerous because, the tip of the Keratome may hit and puncture the anterior capsule and actually tear it. The direction of the keratome is horizontal up to the end of the tunnel, then downwards to cause entry of the tip, then horizontal again to complete the entry incision. If a mistake is made here to push the keratome all the way downwards, without changing the direction, it will hit the lens.

4) The keratome is removed and the anterior chamber is filled with Viscoelastics.

## CLEAR CORNEAL INCISION

In present day Phaco surgery, clear corneal incision is preferred for many reasons. Main reason being that, it is astigmatically neutral and Temporal incision can be given, it is bloodless, painless, can be done with Topical Anesthesia, can be done with preexisting Glaucoma Bleb or in combined surgery and many more advantages.

There are several ways to perform the Clear Corneal Incision; for the sake of simplicity I shall describe one of the most preferred methods.

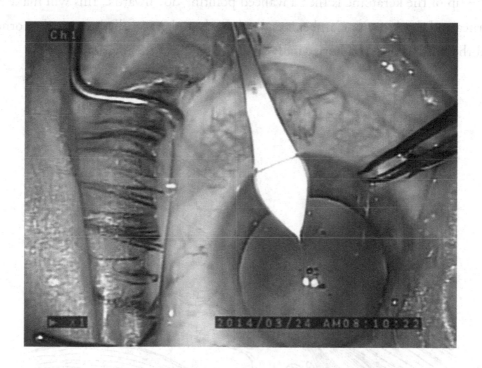

(Fig 12 Clear Corneal Incision with knife: Note that the widest part of the knife has to pass through the incision.)

**Clear Corneal tunnel is done in three easy steps:**

First, a toothed forceps is taken in left hand and Keratome in the right hand.

The Keratome may be 2.8 or 3.1 mm as preferred by the surgeon. With the forceps, the eyeball is fixed and kept steady. The site of the clear corneal incision is next chosen. Usually, the incision site may be anywhere between 1 to 4 O' Clock position for the left eye and 8 to 11 O clock position for the Right eye. The incision site should be just in front of the conjunctival vascular arcade.

**Step 1**) A horizontal groove 300 micron depth is made or just the tip of the keratome is engaged at the site with tip parallel to the corneal epithelium. With counter pressure from the forceps, the cornea is entered.

**Step 2**) the keratome blade is then flattened so that the blade now rests on the sclera and the tip of the keratome is advanced into the corneal stroma for 2 to 2.5 mm. Some keratomes have markings on them how much to enter.

**Step 3**) the tip of the keratome is then advanced pointing downwards. This will make a dimple on the cornea and the Anterior Camber is entered slowly and gracefully keeping the corneal valve intact and the knife is directed horizontally again to complete the incision.

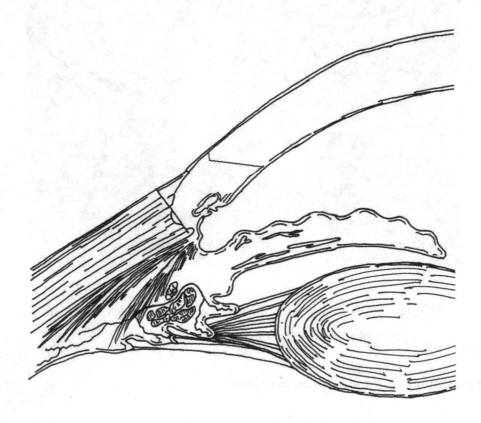

(Fig. 13 Clear corneal incision direction: Note that the direction of
the knife is vertical then horizontal and then again vertical)

**Points to remember:**

a) Once the eye is entered, the blade should be advanced gradually and not to push abruptly which may cause damage to iris or the cornea.

b) A direct push with the keratome will enter the anterior chamber but will not create a three plane self sealing wound.

c) Too short tunnel is formed if the blade is not flattened this and will make the phaco surgery difficult and the incision is not self sealing.

d) Too long tunnel happens if the direction of the Keratome tip is not changed and allowed to go too far into the cornea. This will cause distortion of the cornea when phaco tip is introduced and make the surgery difficult.

e) Lastly, the blade of the Keratome is to be kept parallel to the lens while entering and passing through the A/C otherwise, injury may happen to the lens, iris or the cornea.

Both the Scleral Tunnel and Clear Corneal incisions have advantages and disadvantages.

It is important to decide which type of incision is appropriate for a particular case based on history, type of cataract, hardness of the nucleus and the Patients temperament.

Firstly, Clear Corneal incision has distinctive advantages in patients having bleeding disorders, taking anticoagulants, in cases of Glaucoma whether a combined surgery is performed or having a preexisting bleb, conjunctival scarring and Dry eye syndrome. It is easier and quicker to perform and gives rise to less astigmatism.

The disadvantages are, if not properly closed may cause Infection or endophthalmitis, in case of hard Cataracts, if Conversion to SICS is necessary, it is more difficult to enlarge the incision and gives rise to post operative Astigmatism.

Scleral Tunnel Incision is good for both phaco surgery and SICS. In case of hard cataracts if conversion to SICS or ECCE is necessary, the wound can easily be enlarged without sacrificing sutureless self sealing surgery. It is moderately astigmatically neutral and if not self sealing, one suture can easily be applied. Risk of infection is less because the wound is under the conjunctiva and fully covered.

I prefer clear corneal temporal approach in patients who are cooperative, have Nucleus hardness up to Grade III and good red reflex at microscope and this is the preferred incision in phaco surgery. I prefer Scleral Tunnel Incision in all cases whenever I am performing surgery on Hard Cataracts or I am not sure about the capability of my machine to handle the hardness of the nucleus, I can then easily convert to other procedures of nucleus delivery without compromising the suture less surgery and foldable lens implant. Clear Corneal tunnel surgery is the state of the art in modern Phaco Surgery but the surgeon has to ultimately decide what type of incision will yield best result for the particular patient at the particular situation with particular type of cataract.

In phaco surgery, a good incision is the key to success for an astigmatically neutral sutureless closure of the wound. A blunt keratome should never be used for the incision, if the blades are not cutting, this should be changed immediately. Construction of the incision and the wound is to be practiced very well before entering into the other steps of the surgery.

Although Clear Corneal Tunnel incision is the gold standard in phacoemulsification surgery today, but I feel that, the new surgeons should learn both the types of incisions for cataract surgery. In the developing countries it is essential because, they shall have to operate in many adverse conditions and in many places a phaco machine may not be available. Scleral tunnel if properly constructed, can give very good results in SICS cases. In the developed world, the surgeons should learn both the techniques of incision because if over the years, a patient comes with very hard morgagnian cataract where phacoemulsification would be risky, SICS can be performed and also if the surgeons from developed country travels to a developing country to perform surgeries, where phaco machine is not available, SICS can be performed with a scleral tunnel incision. It is easier to learn these techniques by a young surgeon at the very beginning of the training.

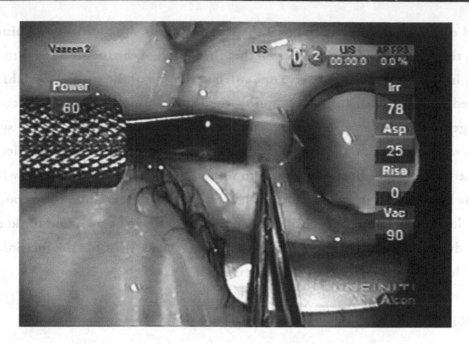

(Fig.14 Clear Corneal incision with Diamond Knife: Note that the knife needs extreme care and the widest part of the knife is the point where measurement is taken)

## Mechanics of Temporal Clear Corneal incision:

It is very important for the surgeon to understand the physics of the temporal clear corneal incision which is the standard incision today for phaco surgery. The temporal incision can be anywhere from 1 to 4 O' clock position or 8 to 11 O' clock depending upon which eye is in question. The entry should be with a 2.8 or a 3.1 keratome. After the 300 Micron horizontal grooves are made, the appropriate keratome is taken and the corneal stroma is entered. Initially, the blade of the keratome rests on the sclera with the tip slightly elevated and advanced in to the corneal stroma for 2.5 to 3 mm inside the cornea. The anterior chamber is entered by dipping the tip of the keratome downwards. Once the A/C is entered, the blade is again made horizontal and the incision is completed. The measurement is important because, if the tunnel is short and is 1.5 mm, a suture placement is necessary to avoid wound leakage. Whereas, if the tunnel is more than 3 mm in length, it is extremely difficult to perform Irrigation and Aspiration of the subincisional cortex. It is important that the surgeon does not tort the wrist or angle the keratome while making the incision otherwise, the roof of the tunnel will be higher on one side and it will not be self sealing. While learning the incision, it is a good idea to measure on the keratome how much a 2.5 mm and a 3mm looks like physically under the microscope.

At the end of this step of phaco surgery the surgeon needs to confirm two points before moving to the next step. First point is, whether the length of the incision is 2.5 to 3 mm or not. Anything less, be prepared to give one stitch at the end of the surgery, anything more, be prepared to have a difficult aspiration of the subincisional cortex. The second point is, the surgeon needs to ensure that the width of the incision will give a good seal of the wound between 2.8 mm to 3.1 mm whatever that is for the phaco needle and sleeve being used. If the width is too short, it will lead to wound burn and if it is too large will lead to continuous leakage and instability of the anterior chamber. Therefore, the keratome is to be chosen depending upon the type of phaco needle which is to be used and the keratome is to be introduced so that the widest part of the keratome passes inside the incision because it is the widest part where the measurement is taken.

## SIDE PORT INCISION:

The side port incision is usually a clear corneal tunnel incision using a 15 degree keratome and is placed two clock hours away from the main incision. Thus if the main incision is at 12 O'clock position, the side port will be at 2 O'clock position. If the incision is at 11 O'clock position, the side port is at 1 O' clock position and so on. The side port should not be too large or it will cause escape of BSS during surgery, or too long which will cause distortion of the cornea. The limbal side port incision should be 1 mm wide and 0.75 mm long. If performing surgery under topical anesthesia, the side port incision is performed first and then the corneal tunnel incision is given. If performing surgery under regional local injection anesthesia, the entry incision is made first and the side port incision is usually made next with the eyeball filled with viscoelastics.

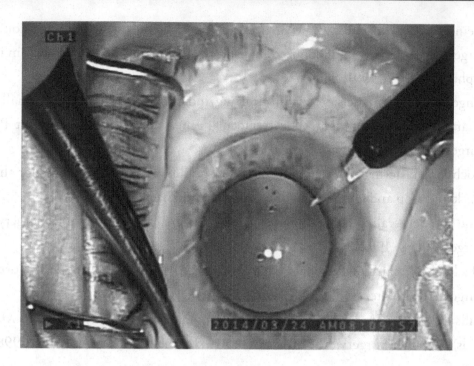

**(Fig.15 Side port Incision: Note that the side port must be at
a comfortable distance from the main incision)**

Before the surgeon makes these two incisions, it is to be ensured that the surgeon places the hands comfortably where there is maximum ability to rotate the instruments inside the eye, so that there is no need to tort the body or hand in order to handle the instruments comfortably inside the anterior chamber of the eye. A very common mistake is to make the two incisions too close or too distant while it becomes difficult to manipulate them throughout the surgery. The distance between the main Phaco incision and the Side Port incision should be around 35 degrees for a small eye ball and 45 degrees for a large eye ball and in between for a standard size eye ball.

## References:

1. Leyland MD. Corneal curvature changes associated with corneal tunnel phacoemulsification. Ophthalmology. 1996; 103:867-88.
2. Fine IH. Self-sealing corneal tunnel incision for small-incision cataract surgery. Ocular Surgery News. 1992.
3. Fine HI. Architecture and construction of a self-sealing incision for cataract surgery. J Cataract Refract Surg. 1991; 17 (Supp): 672-6.

4.  Steinert RF, Brint SF, White SM, et al. Astigmatism after small incision cataract surgery. A prospective, randomized, multi-center comparison of 4 and 6.5 mm incisions. Ophthalmology 11991; 98: 417-24.

5.  Singer JA. Frown incision for minimizing induced astigmatism after small incision cataract surgery with rigid optic intraocular lens implantation. J Cataract Refractive Surgery. 1991; J17(Supp):677-88.

6.  KochPS. Mastering phacoemulsification: A simplified manual strategies for the spring, crack and stop and chop technique, Thorofare NJ: Slack;1994:19.

7.  Fine IH. Self-sealing corneal tunnel incision for small-incision cataract surgery. Ocular Surgery News. 1992.

8.  Mackool RJ. Current Personal Phaco Procedure. In Fine IH (Ed): Clear-Corneal Lens Surgery. Thorofare, NJ: SLACK; 1999; 239-50.

9.  Gills JP, Gayton JL. Reducing pre-existing astigmatism. In Gills JP, Fenzl R, Martin RG (Eds). Cataract Surgery: The State-of-the Art. Thorofare, NJ: SLACK Inc; 1998.

# Chapter 10
# CAPSULORHEXIS

**Anterior Capsule:**

The anterior capsule of the lens has to be removed in order to gain access to the nucleus of the cataract. Removal of the anterior capsule can be done in two ways:

1) Anterior Capsulotomy
2) Anterior Capsulorhexis

**Anterior Capsulotomy can be performed by various techniques:**

A. Beer Can Opener
B. Christmas Tree
C. Circular or triangular
D. D shaped
E. Envelope Technique

Now days it is not necessary to learn these different types of Anterior Capsulotomy. Can Opener Capsulotomy for hard Cataracts in performing SICS and Capsulorhexis in all other cases is now established to be superior to all other techniques.

**Can Opener capsulotomy is discussed in the chapter of Small Incision Cataract Surgery.**

**Anterior Capsulorhexis:**

Capsulorhexis is one of the most important steps of Phaco Surgery up to the extent that, if the Rhexis goes wrong, Phacosurgery should be converted to Small Incision Cataract Surgery (SICS) or, another surgical procedure. Performing anterior chamber phaco has so many complications that, it should better be avoided. A larger incision SICS surgery gives much better surgical outcome than phacoemulsification in the anterior chamber.

**Advantages of Capsulorhexis:**

1. Essential for in the Bag Phacoemulsification surgery.
2. Neat round Capsulorhexis will stand in the bag manipulations of the nucleus without tearing.
3. The bag will withstand pressures of the implanted IOL
4. Clearly visible Capsulorhexis edge facilitates in the bag placement of the IOL
5. Minimum possibility of IOL decentration.
6. Makes it possible to implant specialty lenses like Multifocal or Toric lenses.

**<u>Technique of Capsulorhexis:</u>** There is no right or wrong way to perform anterior Capsulorhexis. A smooth round edge is the most important criterion. The size should be from 5 mm to 5.5 mm round or oval in shape. This can be achieved by using a Cystitome, Capsulorhexis forceps or both the instruments. The clock hours described is taken as an imaginary clock with the point of entry and position of the surgeon as 12 O clock position.

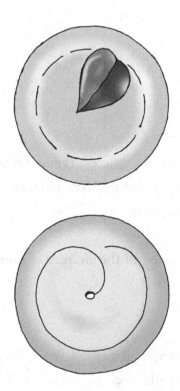

(Fig.16 Direction of capsulorhexis : Note that the direction of rhexis is either clockwise or anti clockwise but the rhexis margin has to come outside in to complete a complete round rhexis with intact margin)

**The following are the prerequisites for a good Capsulorhexis:**

1. The anterior chamber should be filled with enough Viscoelastic to create a positive pressure on the anterior capsule.

2. The centrifugal forces created by the Vitreous pressure must be counteracted by using enough good quality Viscoelastic in the anterior chamber. All misdirection and failure of RHEXIS happens because of mismatch between these two opposing forces. Therefore, as soon as viscoelastic escapes out of the anterior chamber, it must be replaced to create a positive pressure and flatten the anterior capsule.

3. The anterior capsule has to be subjected to tearing forces.

4. The torn anterior capsule must be folded on the intact portion of the anterior capsule for the tear to proceed.

5. Direction of the tear is Centripetal not Centrifugal.

6. The Cystitome gives better anterior chamber stability while the Rhexis forceps gives better grip and tear speed.

7. The pupillary margin can be used as a reference to guide the size and position of the rhexis.

8. It is better to tear in slow turns and to grasp and regrasp the capsule every two clock hour's position at a time, speedy rhexis can be done in expert hands only.

9. The rhexis is to be finished outside to inwards to have a smooth margin.

## CAPSULORHEXIS USING A CYSTITOME:

A bent cystitome is made by bending the tip of a 26 G needle and curving it to give a good grip works well and disposable cystitome is also available.

The entry to the anterior chamber at this point should be small. Viscoelastic is injected at the 6 O clock position and anterior chamber is filled fully.

The cystitome may be attached with to a 3 cc syringe filled with BSS or may be fixed on the tip of the Irrigation line.

Entry to the anterior chamber is important; the end of the needle is sharp and may cause damage to the anterior capsule or the cornea.

111

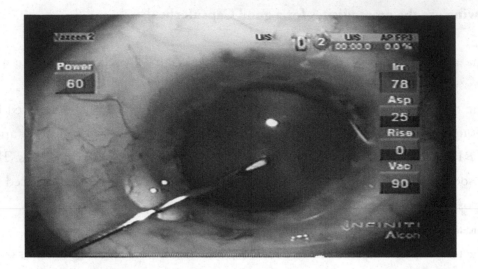

(Fig.17 Start Rhexis with Cystitome : Note that it is a good practice to start
the rhexis with a cystitome and make a cut of 2.5 to 3 mm length)

Hold the syringe or the irrigation line like a pen with hand in pronation; enter the anterior chamber with the tip of the cystitome sideways and horizontal, rotating this in between your thumb and index fingers.

After entering the anterior chamber, rotate the syringe and the cystitome again so that the tip of the cystitome is now pointing towards the anterior capsule. It is very important to have the end of the cystitome visible at all times and not to engage the iris or any other structure while entering the A/C or any other subsequent maneuvers. It is very easy to make injury to the endothelium or iris at this stage.

Advance the needle to the center of the anterior capsule by slightly pronating the wrist with the tip of the cystitome directed downwards. Make a small incision at this position and make a smooth cut in the anterior capsule for about 2.5 mm towards the 9 O clock.

Next important step is to initiate the tear and start by raising a flap of the capsule and folding it onto the intact part of the capsule itself.

It must be remembered that, your hand movements must be soft and deliberate. If you are not gentle to insert the needle, you may end up with a linear cut in the anterior capsule from 12 o clock to 6 O clock positions with the antecedent disadvantages, or you may make injury to the iris or cornea making the surgery difficult.

Once the initial tear is made, the rest of the process is simple. Push to proceed the tear to 7 O clock downwards, then change the direction of the needle in a circular fashion to proceed to 6 and 5 O clock positions. Once 5 O clock position is reached, the direction of the cystitome is to tear upwards centripetally to come to 3 O clock position. Next make a circular motion of the cystitome to 2, 1 and then 12 O clock positions. Next the movement of the cystitome has to change circularly downwards away from you to come to 9 O clock position to meet the original tear outside in to complete the rhexis. Change the direction of the cystitome every clock hour. If the A/C becomes shallow at any point, stop, refill the anterior chamber with Viscoelastic and proceed again. If you cannot see the edge of the rhexis stop and inject Viscoelastic, see the margin and start again in the proper direction. The Capsulorhexis can be started at any convenient clock hour position as the surgeon wants. It can be started at 3 O clock position and done clockwise and come back to 3 O clock position to complete.

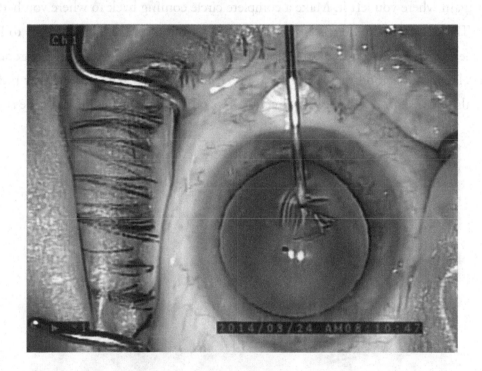

(Fig.18 Capsulorhexis with Cystitome : Note that the whole
rhexis may be completed with the Cystitome)

It is hard to do rhexis on a soft cataract or in presence of a liquid cortex in hyper mature cataract. This needs caution and use of a dye to stain the anterior capsule.

## CAPSULORHEXIS USING UTTARATA FORCEPS:

Approach to perform rhexis with Rhexis forceps is different. Fill the Anterior chamber with good viscoelastic preferably Healon or its equivalent. Hold the forceps in your Right hand in between thumb and index fingers and balanced on the middle finger. Introduce the forceps with the tip closed into the A/C, aim to go to the center. Make a point tear at the center and using the forceps and tear a small corner or "Ear" of the capsule. Grasp the ear and initiate the tear toward 8 O clock or 9 O clock position and continue tear in anticlockwise direction making a circular movement to 6 O clock position. Next grasp the edge of the rhexis again and pull laterally and upward direction to come to 4 O clock position and continue the tear in a circular fashion releasing and re grasping the edge of the rhexis every two clock hours. If the edge of the rhexis is not visible or if Viscoelastic has escaped, remove the forceps carefully from the A/C, inject Viscoelastic and start the rhexis again where you left it. Make a complete circle coming back to where you had started the rhexis. The point to note here is that, Rhexis is not a blind procedure; you have to keep the edge and the end of the rhexis in clear vision all the time. Good Microscope light, good optics, good Viscoelastic and a good rhexis forceps are very important for having a circular rhexis. The rhexis can also be performed clockwise direction depending upon the comfort of the surgeon.

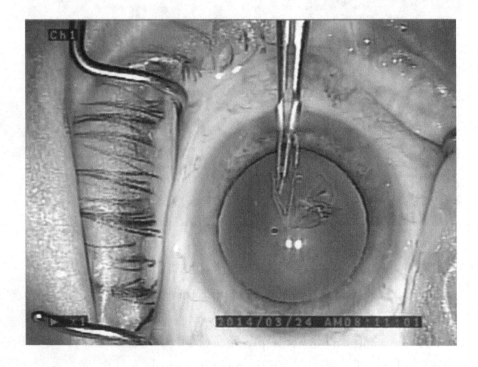

(Fig.19 Capsulorhexis with Forceps: Note that the forceps may be used to perform the whole procedure or may be used in combination with the Cystitome)

**TWO HANDED TECHNIQUE: (For the Beginning surgeon)**

Two handed procedure also works very well for the beginner surgeon who has to balance the hands to hold the torn delicate ear of the anterior capsule and tear this with a circular movement. With the dominant hand hold the forceps and grasp the ear of the rhexis margin and with the other non dominant hand hold the body of the forceps and move the hands harmoniously in a circular fashion as described before, to get a perfect Circular Capsulorhexis. This gives better stabilization of the hands and good outcome.

## Combined Cystitome and Forceps Method

It may be easier to initiate the rhexis with a cystitome, make a cut in the capsule towards the 9 O clock position start the tear with a sweeping motion of the cystitome and fold the torn edge of the capsule continue the rhexis to 6 O clock position as described. It is then easy to grasp the edge of the tear with the forceps and continue the rhexis to complete to 9 O clock position.

I find it most difficult to perform rhexis from 12 O clock to 9 O clock position and prefer to do this part with forceps.

**It is not possible to teach Capsulorhexis by any written description, there is no right or wrong way of doing it. One has to practice to make it perfect every time before any other step of phaco surgery is performed.**

## Dye assisted Capsulorhexis

Dye staining of the anterior capsule is one of the most important advances in the management of complicated cataracts. Several dye has been used to stain the anterior capsule 1998, Horiguchi first published the use of 0.5% indocyanine green (ICG) to stain the anterior capsule, in 1999, Melles described the use of 0.1% Trypan blue dye to stain the anterior capsule.

Presently, 0.1 % or 0.06 % Trypan Blue is universally used to stain the anterior capsule for Capsulorhexis of hyper- mature or mature cataracts where a red reflex is difficult to obtain.

For an Ophthalmologist in developing countries, it is very important to learn Dye assisted anterior Capsulorhexis.

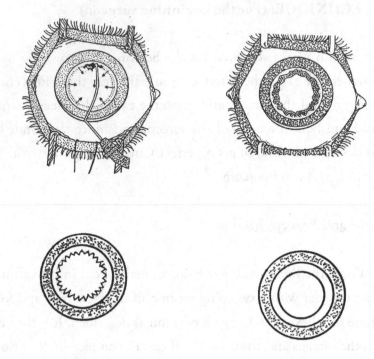

Fig 20: ( Different types of capsulotomy in SICS)

## Indications:

1. White Hypermature Cataract
2. Whenever cataract is mature enough where red reflex is absent
3. Cataracts with dense white cortical spokes where a uniform red reflex is difficult to obtain, the underlying nucleus may not be hard.
4. Pediatric cataracts or cataracts in young people.
5. During training period, it may be useful to use the dye in all cataracts because; the young surgeon will have better visibility of the capsule and will learn capsulorhexis easily.
6. Complicated Cataracts

## Staining technique:

Different surgeons use the dye to stain the anterior capsule in different ways. The following is the most practiced method:

116

The dye is injected under sterilized air introduced into the anterior chamber. After staining the anterior capsule, the air is replaced with viscoelastics and rhexis is performed with cystitome or uttarata forceps as required.

1. One way to obtain sterile air is to fill the syringe within the plastic sterile packet as far as possible to obtain sterile air which is present inside the packet. This technique is simple. Take a disposable syringe and before opening the packet, pull the plunger as far as it can go inside the unopened packet, usually it is possible to get 0.5 ml sterile air to suck up in the syringe, then open the packet and use the air.

2. The other way to obtain sterile air is little difficult. Take a sterile disposable syringe out of the packet, hold the syringe and burn the tip of the needle on the flame of a spirit lamp. When it is red hot, bring it away and pull the plunger to fill it up with air. The air will pass through the hot needle and make it sterile. Leave the whole syringe in this position on the instrument table for some time until the air cools down which will take about 5 minutes.

3. Now change the needle with a 30 G air cannula and introduce the air through the side port incision to fill up the anterior chamber.

4. Take the Trypan Blue dye in a tuberculin syringe fitted with a 30 G cannula.

5. Place several drops of the dye on the anterior capsule beneath the air bubble.

6. Wait for one or two minutes and wash the dye out with BSS in a syringe fitted with a 30 G cannula.

7. The anterior chamber is next filled with viscoelastic and the rhexis is performed with Cystitome, Uttarata forceps or combination of both as described earlier.

8. Some surgeons prefer to fill the anterior chamber with cohesive viscoelastics and introduce the dye beneath the blob of viscoelastic partition. In this method, the capsule takes up more of the stain and stains better. The technique with air bubble is simple but the surface tension of the air bubble displaces some of the Trypan blue and the anterior capsule gets less stained.

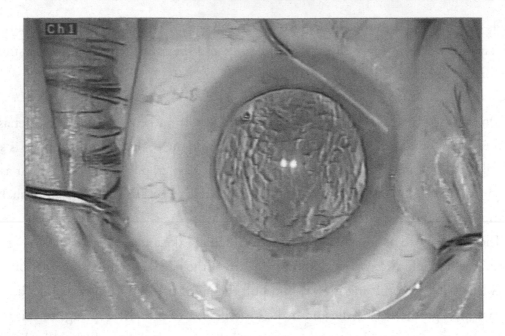

Fig. 21: (Introduction of viscoelastic in to the A/C)

## Misdirected Capsulorhexis

Management of misdirected Capsulorhexis is a challenge to the surgeon. The following are a few suggestions how to salvage a misdirected Capsulorhexis.

1.  If after initiation of the rhexis it tends to tear towards the periphery or in other words, run away, one has to recognize the situation and immediately stop the rhexis at this position.

2.  Start the rhexis at the opposite site and come back to the original site to complete the rhexis. Suppose, you started the rhexis at 9 O' clock position and planned to go anticlockwise, but it started to run away at 7 O' clock position, stop, refill the anterior chamber with viscoelastic, come back to 9 O' clock position raise a small ear of the intact edge of the capsule in the opposite direction and proceed in a clockwise direction and come clockwise to 7 O clock position and continue the rhexis clockwise past 7 O' cock position to come back to 9 O' clock position, and will need to make a slightly bigger size rhexis.

3.  If you cannot raise an ear of the anterior capsule at 9 O'clock position, extend the anterior capsule cut to 3 O' Clock position horizontally and make two rhexis. 3 to 7 O' Clock in the clockwise direction and 3 to 9 O' clock in anticlockwise direction.

4.  Do the rhexis from 9 O clock position in counterclockwise direction up to 7 O clock position to meet the previous margin of the rhexis and this is easier to do with the forceps.

5. If you started the rhexis cut from the center horizontally towards the 9 O clock but cannot raise the initial flap to start the tearing which may happen in more elastic capsules, take an angled Vannas scissors, make a cut at the margin of the initial cut to raise an "ear" of the capsule and proceed with the rhexis with forceps or cystitome and when coming back to complete the rhexis you have to come outside in to make it round or oval making sure that the margin is intact.

It is very important to remember that, if a rhexis starts to extend to periphery, the pressure in the anterior chamber has to be increased by using enough viscoelastics and a positive pressure is maintained throughout the procedure. Shallowing of the A/C is dangerous at this situation and slow rhexis with repeated injection of Viscoelastic like viscoat is preferred.

## Causes of complications in Capsulorhexis:

There are several factors that are responsible for failure to obtain a good Capsulorhexis:

1. Poor red reflex: This may be due to Mature and Hypermature cataracts, Small pupil, bad microscope illumination, corneal epithelial injury due to repeated topical application of drops, Vitreous opacity and corneal edema.
2. Sudden Eye Movement: This may be due to inadequate anesthesia and sudden movement of the head or eyes during Capsulorhexis may cause misdirection.
3. Shallowing of the Anterior Chamber: This may be due to preexisting shallow anterior chamber or due to back vitreous pressure.
4. Age of the patient: The younger the patient, the more elastic the anterior capsule is and it may be difficult to make a rhexis in young patients with elastic capsule.

## Prevention of Misdirection of Capsulorhexis:

The surgeon can take certain preventive measures to avoid run away of the rhexis.

1) Deep Anterior chamber is to be maintained at all times. This can be done using good quality viscoelastic and replacing the viscoelastic frequently as it escapes from the A/C.
2) Reduction of Intraocular Pressure by Acetazolamide in the morning of the surgery.
3) Dilate the pupil well and in small pupil cases, use of appropriate instruments to keep the pupil dilated.

4) In difficult cases, slow rhexis grasping the capsule every clock hours can help to keep the rhexis round.

5) In difficult cases, it may be better to create a smaller Capsulorhexis and enlarge the same later on.

6) Check the Microscope to clean the optics and a good red reflex at the start of the surgery.

7) If the red reflex is poor or obscured for any reason, use Trypan Blue for staining the capsule and proceed with caution.

Having said these points, I want to remind that, it is not easy to retrieve a runaway rhexis. Use of a good viscoelastic is the key to successful Capsulorhexis and will be very easy if you remember that, the pressure in the anterior chamber has be more that the Intralenticular and vitreous pressure. In Hypermature cataracts, Acetazolamide and or Mannitol will reduce the vitreous pressure, also use of good viscoelastic like Healon GV, or Viscoat will aid in performing good Capsulorhexis.

If it becomes difficult and beyond your control to get a capsulorhexis, don't allow the rhexis tear to run to the posterior capsule and cause posterior capsule tear. Perform a can opener capsulotomy and convert to SICS. This is much better to have an intact Posterior capsule to implant a Posterior Chamber IOL than to have a run - away rhexis and to tear past the zonules to posterior capsule to make the surgery more complicated. If the rhexis margin has gone beyond your sight, stop and review the situation, take the best and prudent decision, but don't panic or rush the surgery. Remember that, a 7 mm incision SICS with can opener capsulotomy with intact posterior capsule, a posterior chamber lens implanted and four stitches placed is a much better option than a torn posterior capsule, nucleus drop or an A/C IOL implant.

**Summary of Capsulorhexis:**

**Capsulorhexis is the single most important step of phaco surgery without which in the bag phacoemulsification is compromised with the consequences. Capsulorhexis ensures better refractive outcome, better hydrodissection, rotation of the nucleus and less chance of zonular tear. The consensus now is to create a Capsulorhexis that is 0.5 mm to 1 mm smaller than the optic size of the IOL to be implanted. Thus, if the IOL optic is 6mm in diameter, the rhexis should be 5 to 5.5 mm and if the optic size is 7 mm, the rhexis size should be 6 mm. This gives the best refractive outcome. Therefore, the surgeon must know the optic size of the IOL before performing the**

rhexis. Although there are many ways to perform the rhexis as described, it is safer to use the combined cystitome and forceps method. After filling the anterior chamber with viscoelastic first enter the eye with a cystitome and make a horizontal cut on the anterior capsule for about 2.5 mm to 3 mm radius from the center and therefore imagine that when it goes all the way round it will give a 5 mm to 6 mm diameter rhexis. Now lift the edge of the cut to make a little lip and bring the cystitome out. Next enter the eye with the Uttarata forceps and grab the lip to initiate the tear and proceed in a circular fashion grasping and re grasping the edge of the rhexis every 2 clock hours. This will give a controlled circular Capsulorhexis margin and as the surgeon gets experienced, the clock hour may be extended. While grasping the edge of the capsular tear every two clock hours remember to hold at the base of the tear, not at the apex of it. Note that, if you create a small Capsulorhexis you run the risk of developing a capsular contraction and a myopic shift while a big rhexis will give a tilted lens and hyperopic shift in the post operative period. If the rhexis is compromised, it is important to recognize this and take appropriate corrective measures to overcome the misdirection. In two handed technique, the surgeon can control the movement of the forceps with both hands and thus creating a round margin is ensured. The procedure has to be repeated again and again before proficiency is gained and whatever method is used, a round rhexis is to be ensured each time and every time.

## REFERENCES :

1. Gimbel HV, Neuhann T. Development, advantages, and methods of the continuous circular capsulorhexis technique. J Cataract Refract Surg. 1990;16:31-37.

2. Melles G, de Waard P, Pameyer J, Beekhuis W. Trypan blue capsule staining to visualize the capsulorhexis in cataract surgery. J Cataract Refract Surg. 1999;25:7-9.

3. Fritz W. Fluorescein blue light-assisted capsulorhexis for mature or hypermature cataract. J Cataract Refract Surg. 1998;24:19-20.

4. Kayikicioglu O, Erakgun T, Guler C. Trypan blue mixed with sodium hyaluronate for capsulorhexis (letter). J Cataract Refract Surg. 2001;27:970.

5. Horiguchi M, Miyake K, Ohta I, Ito Y. Staining of the lens capsule for circular continuous capsulorhexis in eyes with white cataract. Arch Ophthalmol. 1998;116:535-537.

6. Chang D. Capsule staining and mature cataracts: A comparison of indocyanine green and trypan blue dyes. Video report. Br J Ophthalmol. 2000;84

7.  Newsom TH, Oetting TN. Indocyanine green staining in traumatic cataract. J Cataract Refract Surg. 2000;26:1691-1693.

8.  Chang D. Capsule staining and mature cataracts: A comparison of indocyanine green and trypan blue dyes. Video report. Br J Ophthalmol. 2000;84(August).

9.  Chang DF. Clinical comparison of ICG and trypan blue due for mature cataract. Paper presented at: annual meeting of the American Society of Cataract and Refractive Surgery; April 28-May 2, 2001; San Diego, Calif.

10. Wakabayashi T, Yamamoto N. Posterior capsule staining and posterior continuous curvilinear capsulorrhexis in congenital cataract. *J Cataract Refract Surg.* 2002;28:2042-2044.

11. Dada VK, Sharma N, Pangtey MS, et al. Comparison of various anterior capsular staining methods for capsulorrhexis in white cataracts. Paper presented at: annual meeting of the American Academy of Ophthalmology; November 11-14, 2001; New Orleans, La.

12. Saini JS, Jain AK, Sukhija J, et al. Anterior and posterior capsulorrhexis in pediatric cataract surgery with or without trypan blue dye: Randomized prospective clinical study. *J Cataract Refract Surg.* 2003;29:1733-1737.

13. De Waard PW, Budo CJ, Melles GR. Trypan blue capsular staining to "find" the leading edge of a "lost" capsulorrhexis. *Am J Ophthalmol.* 2002;134:271-272.

14. Singh AJ, Sarodia UA, Brown L, et al. A histological analysis of lens capsules stained with trypan blue for capsulorrhexis in phacoemulsification cataract surgery. *Eye.* 2003;17:567-570

15. Akahoshi T. Mixing a viscoelastic and a capsular dye. *Cataract & Refractive Surgery Today.* 2005;March:39-46.

16. Marques DM, Marques FF, Osher RH. Three-step technique for staining the anterior lens capsule with indocyanine green or trypan blue. *J Cataract Refract Surg.* 2004;30:13-16.

# Chapter 11

# HYDRODISSECTION__AND_ HYDRODELINEATION

Hydrodissection is one of the most important steps in phacoemulsification. The new surgeon must take time in this step and once again, not to proceed to the next step until a good hydrodissection and rotation of the nucleus is achieved. Poor result may happen due to poor hydrodissection and lack of rotation of the nucleus. Forceful rotation due to incomplete hydrodissection will cause Zonular Dehiscence and a difficult surgery.

Hydrodissection means passage of fluid between epinucleus and the capsule by which a fluid wave separates the epinucleus including the rest of the lens from the capsule. The fluid essentially frees the nucleus including epinucleus from the capsule.

Hydrodelineation involves passage of fluid wave between the firmer epinucleus and endonucleus. In actual fact, passage of fluid between the nucleus any other part of the lens is hydrodelineation. It can separate the Nucleus and Cortex, the Epinucleus and Cortex, loosen the cortex and in this way, every time you pass a fluid wave, some plane separates from the nucleus and the nucleus becomes freer. By this statement I am not encouraging to go on doing hydro procedures, rather to make it understandable that passage of fluid wave in between the different planes of the lens is important.

**The effects produced by the hydro procedures are:**

1) Rotation of the Endonucleus
2) Rotation of the Epinucleus
3) Loosening of the cortex

During phacoemulsification, the phaco tip cannot be moved around the anterior chamber except in tortional handpiece. In most machines it works from one place, the center of the anterior chamber (A/C). Therefore, the nucleus has to be mobile and rotated to bring the fragments to the phaco tip for it to catch and emulsify the same. Hydro procedures make the nucleus mobile,thus helps to rotate it, flip it, break it and helps to bring the broken parts to the phaco tip for emulsification.

After good hydrodissection and hydrodelineation, it is easy to remove the endonucleus leaving behind the epinucleus and the cortex which protects the posterior capsule.

The epinucleus is then removed with low phaco power and held with higher vacuum.

The cortex is next aspirated by Irrigation and Aspiration at high vacuum and needs no phaco power.

## TECHNIQUE OF HYDRODISSECTION:

A 2 cc syringe is taken and filled with BSS and fitted with a right angle 27 G cannula. Other types of hydrodissection cannula are also available. A slightly flattened tip to deliver a fan like jet of fluid is preferred. Autoclaved Glass Syringe give smooth movement, a plastic disposable syringe gives better sterility. Tactile feedback is the same with both the types of the syringe.

First, a small amount of viscoelastic is expressed out of the anterior chamber, and this is important to allow the viscoelastic to escape so that, there is enough space in the anterior chamber to make the dissection possible.

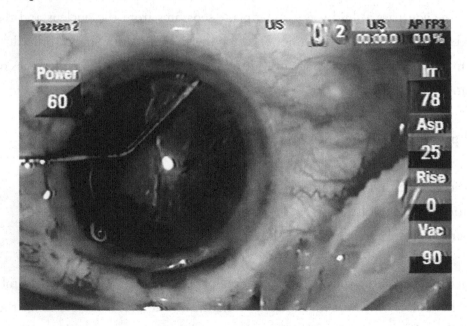

(Fig 22 A : Hydrodissection : Note that the fluid wave must propagate below the nucleus)

The tip of the cannula is introduced just beneath the anterior capsule. The cannula not only hooks the Capsulorhexis edge but also lifts the anterior capsule slightly upwards. This makes it more likely that the hydrostatic wave will follow the inside of the capsule. Since the volume of fluid that can be injected into the capsular bag is limited, a small-diameter cannula (e.g., 30 gauge or 27 gauge) should be used. The increased flow resistance from a smaller cannula maximizes the hydrostatic force that can be generated by a relatively small volume of fluid. The most effective fluid jet is one that is brief, sufficiently forceful, and oriented in a radial direction.

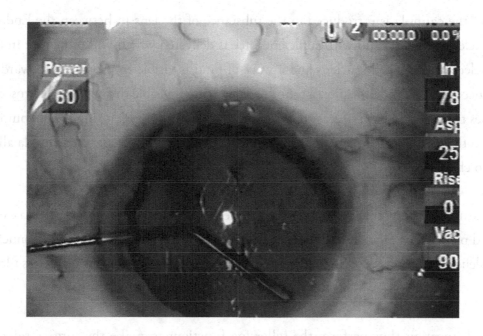

(Fig.23 B Hydrodissection : Note the flow or BSS with a right angle cannula)

A small jet of fluid is injected and the fluid produces a slowly propagating wave that has scalloped advancing borders because it is passing through the cortex as it hugs the inner capsular surface.

Viewing the fluid wave is the most important thing. If the fluid wave is not visible, the nucleus is compressed by pressing on the shaft of the cannula and the fluid is allowed to escape. Hydrodissection through another site is next tried. Repeated trial is continued until a propagating fluid wave is visible, and the hydrodissection is complete. It is important to remember that too forceful a fluid jet may propagate very quickly breaking the posterior capsule and too slow a fluid wave will not dissect at all. The fluid wave must have sufficient hydrostatic force to dissect through the path of greatest resistance. This force must be generated quickly because there is a limited volume of fluid that can be safely injected. Overtly tentative and gradual injection may empty the syringe, but only produce circulation of balanced salt solution within the anterior chamber. Therefore balance of the force of fluid delivery is very important to practice.

## HYDRODELINEATION

If proper hydrodissection is achieved, hydrodelineation is not a must. Hydrodelineation frees off the endonucleus from the epinucleus and makes it easy to be removed by less phaco energy.

The Tip of the cannula is introduced in the substance of the lens in between the Endonucleus and Epinucleus. A jet of fluid with sufficient force is delivered which will propagate in between the epinucleus and the endonucleus and a wave of fluid is visible to propagate forward. At the end of a successful hydrodelineation a round Golden Ring is visible through the microscope. The fluid passes through the path of least resistance. Sometimes the golden ring is not complete and delineation through another plane may be required. In very soft nucleus, the cannula allows the surgeon to choose

an epinuclear shell of any thickness and hydrodelineation can be performed to make a cleavage at the desired plane. This procedure divides the nucleus circumferentially into an endonucleus and an epinucleus, provides a protective cushion for safe removal of the nucleus using less ultrasound energy.

The hydrodelineation thus perform the following functions to make the surgery safer: 1) The endonucleus and an epinuclear shell are separated. 2) The portion to the nucleus to be removed by phacoemulsification is reduced. 3) Provides a protective cushion which keeps capsule safe during phaco maneuvers. 4) Hydrodelineation is possible in softer nuclei and not possible in a hard nucleus.

## CORTICAL CLEAVING HYDRODISSECTION:

After hydrodissection and hydrodelineation performed, it is easy to emulsify the Nucleus, which rotates within the protective shell of the Epinucleus, requiring less energy. But after that, two important jobs remain waiting. Firstly the Epinucleus which may be bulky has to be removed by the phaco needle. Secondly, the cortical mater has to be stripped from the capsule and removed using the Irrigation and Aspiration handpiece.

Dr. Howard Fine came forward with a unique technique, Cortical Cleaving Hydrodissection. If the procedure can be performed properly, it makes the process of cataract removal by phacoemulsification less time consuming.

## TECHNIQUE:

The hydrodissection cannula is introduced just below the anterior capsule and the anterior capsular flap is lifted away from the cortical mater and the tip of the cannula is advanced very gently as far as possible towards the equator. The cannula maintains the tented up position of the capsule prior to injection of the fluid. Hydration of the cortex prior to reaching the accurate plane between the capsule and the cortex has to be avoided. Because premature hydration of the cortex will direct the fluid wave in wrong direction and some cortex will remain attached to the capsule.

Once the correct plane is reached, a continuous gentle irrigation of a jet of fluid is performed. The fluid wave moves forward and a visible fluid wave is seen under the nucleus propagating around the equator completely separating and cleaving the cortex from the capsule and separates all the adhesions, between the capsule and the cortex, and when this is completed, the nucleus lifts up a little. The injection of fluid must be stopped at this point and the nucleus is decompressed using the shaft of the cannula which usually completes cortical cleaving Hydrodissection. The nucleus can be freely rotated using the cannula or the second instrument.

When Phacoemulsification of the nucleus is performed subsequently, the whole nucleus, epinucleus and the cortical mater are removed together, leaving behind very little cortical mater to be removed by Irrigation and aspiration. Thus the surgical time is reduced and the nucleus can be mobilized and rotated easily without any stress on the zonules.

Cortical cleaving hydrodissection loosens the cortex so that it can be mobilized in large sheets, rather than in thin adherent strips. This enhances the efficiency and safety of cortical removal.

However, in Posterior Subcapsular Cataract, Posterior polar cataract and where Cortico-capsular adhesions are present, my preference is to perform Hydrodelineation and separate hydrodissection rather than Cortical Cleaving Hydrodissection because of the risk of breaking the Posterior capsule with the force of the fluid which has to traverse the space between the capsule and the cortex breaking these adhesions rendering the posterior capsule vulnerable. Hydrodelineation is safer in these situations because it leaves behind a cortical shell which is protective to the posterior capsule during the phacoemulsification of the nucleus.

**INSIDE OUT HYDRODELINEATION** as described by Dr. Abhay Vasavada is a very clever way to hydro delineate the nucleus at the correct plane where the surgeon wants the fluid wave to pass. This requires a central core or trench to be sculpted first before hydrodelineation and then the surgeon goes through the trench to insert a 90 degree bent cannula to hydrodelineate at the correct plane where the surgeon wants to hydrodelineate the nucleus. This keeps a cushion of epinucleus of a desired thickness to protect the capsule. This form of hydrodissection is most important in Posterior polar cataracts and is fully described in chapter 20 D. Please refer to the full article of Dr. Vasavada for details of the procedure.

## POINTS TO BE NOTED FOR PROPER HYDRO PROCEDURES :

Although hydrodissection and hydrodelineation are very important steps in cataract surgery, they are also very delicate steps.

**A. Viscoelastic in the anterior chamber**: This may exert counter pressure and resistance for the fluid wave to pass and Hydro procedures will be difficult. Some viscoelastic must be removed from the anterior chamber before hydro procedures and this is often overlooked.

**B. Block at the Capsulorhexis Margin:** With proper hydrodissection, the nucleus will elevate forward from the posterior capsule. A larger nucleus may rise enough so that it internally blocks the Capsulorhexis opening. Continuing to inject fluid that cannot escape the capsular bag may over inflate the bag and rupture the posterior capsule. If the nucleus suddenly elevates above the hydrodissection wave, the irrigation of fluid must be stopped immediately and the nucleus should be depressed posteriorly with the shaft of cannula to decompress the fluid which is allowed to escape from the nucleus through the Capsulorhexis opening.

**C. Force of the fluid injection**: The fluid wave must have sufficient hydrostatic force to dissect through the path of greatest resistance. This force must be generated quickly and steadily for the fluid to pass through the lens material dissecting it and separating the Endonucleus from the Capsule or Cortex.

If proper hydrodissection is achieved, phaco surgery subsequent steps become easier and can be performed quickly.

If proper hydrodissection or hydrodelineation is not achieved, phacoemulsification becomes a difficult surgery and may become a nightmare for the surgeon.

However, surgery is possible without any hydrodissection or hydrodelineation procedures but this exerts stress on the zonules. In case the hydrodissection fluid wave is not visible during the procedure, the surgeon must be alert not to exert stress on the zonules and minimize surge during surgery.

## References :

1.  Fine IH. Cortical cleaving hydrodissection. J Cataract Refract Surg. 1992;18(5):508-12.
2.  Anis A. Understanding hydrodelineation: The term and related procedures. Ocular Surg News 1991 ;9:134-7.
3.  Faust KJ. Hydrodissection of soft nuclei. Am Intraocular Implant SocJ. 1984;10:75-7
4.  Sheperd JR. In situ fracture. J Cataract Refract Surg. 1990;16:436-40.
5.  Gimbel HV. Divide and conquer nucleofractis phacoemulsification:Development and variations. J Cataract Refract Surg. 1991;17:281-91.
6.  Fine IH. The chip and flip phacoemulsification technique. J Cataract Refract Surg. 1991; 17:366-71.
7.  Fine IH. The choo-choo chop and flip phacoemulsification technique. Operative Techniques in Cataract and Refractive Surgery. 1998;l(2):61-5.
8.  Vasavada AR, Raj SM. Inside-Out delineation. Journal of Cataract Refract Surgery. 2004;30:1167-9.

# Chapter 12
# PHACOEMULSIFICATION AND REMOVAL OF THE NUCLEUS

The phaco surgery is all about bringing out the 12 mm nucleus out through a 3 mm or smaller incision. This is accomplished by breaking up and liquefying the nucleus so that it can be aspirated through a 1 mm diameter Phaco needle. The technique requires several maneuvers to mobilize the nucleus in small fragments, emulsify the fragments and at the same time suck the emulsified material through the needle and phaco handpiece with irrigation and aspiration force.

We know that Cataract is opacification of the Crystaline Lens and this opaque lens must be removed keeping the clear posterior capsule intact through the smallest incision possible. The mechanisms applied to accomplish this depends upon the consistency of the nucleus, its size and capability of the equipment used perform the job.

We come across different types of cataracts with different levels of difficulty to remove it. I did not find two cataracts exactly identical and therefore, every type of cataract deserves special attention.

According to the consistency of the nucleus we come across the following types cataracts:

1. Posterior subcapsular cataract with soft nucleus
2. Grade I Nucleus : slight grey or Greenish Yellow nucleus
3. Grade 2 Nucleus : Yellow colored Nucleus
4. Grade 3 Nucleus : Amber colored nucleus
5. Grade 4 Nucleus : Brown colored nucleus
6. Grade 5 Nucleus: Morganian, Black in color very hard cataract.
7. Hypermature Cataract: Milky White in color Liquid cortex, nucleus hard and sinks down.
8. Fibrotic Cataract : The capsule becomes fibrotic, nucleus is of amber or brown color and hard

The phacoemulsification of these different types of nucleus will depend upon the type of the cataract encountered and the capabilities of machine used. Phacoemulsification is possible in all types of cataract if the surgeon has the understanding about the machine and the type of the cataract he is handling. The machine actually acts like a pet to the surgeon, and will operate the way he or she wants it. The surgeon must decide which type of nucleus is encountered and what will be the best procedure to perform in order to remove the nucleus through a phaco needle 1 mm in diameter and a 2.8 mm or 3 mm incision.

**There are four factors:**

1. Breaking the nucleus in small fragments.
2. Converting these small fragments into liquid using ultrasound power to emulsify the hard nuclear material.
3. Aspiration of the emulsified material.
4. Surge control by the machine or by the surgeon.

Some machines are more efficient than the other in these modalities, but ultimately it is the surgeon who has to make this happen.

Several techniques have been described to perform phacoemulsification and a generalization of the techniques is not possible. Each technique has to be learned and practiced by the operating surgeon and applied judiciously while performing the surgery on a particular patient. The surgeon has to decide which technique will work best for the particular case at the given circumstances. We will therefore describe each technique separately and urge the surgeon to understand the mechanics of each of them and apply it when appropriate.

The following Techniques have been described to perform emulsification of the nucleus:

1. Chip and Flip Technique
2. Divide and Conquer Technique
3. Four Quadrant Divide and Conquer Technique
4. Phaco Chop
5. Stop and Chop
6. Stop Chop and Stuff
7. Bevel Down Phaco chop

Each of these techniques has been described and practiced by renowned surgeons and there are names attached to each technique. For further reading, the surgeon is advised to read the original articles or text books written by the authors who have originally described the procedure. The different techniques described in the next few pages are to assist the surgeon to understand the different procedures to complete the task of nucleus removal.

**Chip and Flip Technique**

The chip and Flip phacoemulsification technique is first described by Dr. I Howard Fine. The other name of the technique is "Spring Surgery".

This is the most effective method of phacoemulsification in soft nucleus.

In this technique, CCC is done; proper hydrodelineation is performed to create a cleavage between the endonucleus and the epinucleus. Hydrodissection is performed to free the cortex and the epinucleus from the capsule. The important part is to perform a good hydrodelineation and reduce the size of the endonucleus. The endonucleus is surrounded by the epinuclear shell along with cortex.

The phacoemulsification is started with low vacuum and low phaco power settings. A central groove is created with caution because in soft cataract cutting is quick and without much resistance. If the nucleus is firm enough to be rotated, groove is continued in the other half of the nucleus. Otherwise if the nucleus is soft and cannot be rotated, a crater is made in the center of the nucleus to create a space for the nucleus to be flipped.

**Next is chipping**, this is done with vacuum setting at 100 or 120 mm and phaco power set to low around 60 to 70. A small part of the nucleus is chipped and brought to the center to emulsify. This leaves a partly chipped endonucleus within the shell of the epinucleus and attached cortex. The nucleotomy made by chipping leaves the rest of the nucleus in protective shell and when held with vacuum and pulled towards the center the whole nucleus flips over and come to the phaco tip easily to be emulsified.

Next move is to hold the side of the nucleus with vacuum at foot position 2 and flipped over. Once the nucleus is free and flips over, bring it to the center at the iris plane and emulsify this by impaling the nucleus at the phaco tip with the second instrument.

Once the nucleus is removed, what are left behind are epinucleus and the cortical shell. It is more difficult to remove the epinucleus. The phaco tip is used to hold the epinucleus at foot position 2 by using occlusion and vacuum only and pulled to the center and a small piece will be emulsified. The rest of the epinucleus is now rotated and flipped to bring to the center and emulsified using low, intermittent phaco power.

If the hydrodissection is good, the cortex will also come with it. The most difficult part of the procedure is to bring the sub incisional cortex and epinucleus to the phaco tip. This is done by dislodging the cortical piece using the second instrument and the piece is rotated to the center and emulsified.

The remaining cortical mater is removed by the I/A handpiece and the tip is used to hold the cortical strands and pulled and striped to the center to be sucked out. If a small amount of cortex is present at the subincisional area, this can be removed after insertion of the IOL and inserting the I/A tip through the side port or using the j cannula for irrigation and aspiration.

This procedure is good for soft cataract where cracking of the nucleus is not possible and also for moderately hard cataract where flipping of the nucleus is possible. The technique involves chipping a part of the nucleus and then flipping it over and held to be emulsified. The epinucleus is also flipped to be emulsified. Extreme caution is to be observed to keep the posterior capsule intact while doing the Irrigation and aspiration of the residual cortex.

Insertion of IOL is performed as in any other method of nucleus removal is employed which will be discussed in a subsequent chapter.

### Divide and conquer technique

The divide and conquer technique is described by DR. Howard Gimbel.

There are actually two different approaches:

1. Trench divide and conquer
2. Crater divide and conquer

The essence of this technique is to create a central space at the middle of the nucleus. The nucleus is then broken into pieces and brought to this center to be emulsified. All other Chopping principles developed later on works basically on this principle.

In soft cataracts, we can flip the nucleus but in harder nuclei it is not possible to flip the harder and bigger nucleus.

### Creating the trench:

After CCC and hydro procedures are completed, the eye is filled with viscoelastics and phaco needle is inserted. A trench is then sculpted from the center to the visible periphery of the nucleus by repeated pass of the tip. The center of the nucleus is thicker than the periphery. Therefore, while sculpting at the center the tip is held vertically down and coming slightly up with the phaco tip when going to the periphery. Dr. Gimbel has described "Down-slope Sculpting" which is a clever way for sculpting the nucleus. The width of the trench should be two phaco tips wide and three phaco tips deep and the red glow is visible at the bottom of the trench.

Next rotate the nucleus 360 degrees and bring the created trench at 12 O clock position and continue to make the trench at the other portion of the nucleus. Thus a trench from 12 O clock position to the 6 O clock position is made. The red glow should be visible at the floor of the trench.

Instead of creating the trench, a crater can be made at the center of the nucleus.

**Cracking:**

Cracking the nucleus is the next step. This can be done in many ways:

1. The phaco tip is buried in one half of the nucleus and a second instrument like spatula is engaged on the other half of the nucleus and the two are separated to opposite directions and the crack is achieved.
2. One curved spatula is introduced through the main incision, one 1.5 mm blunt chopper in introduced through the side port. The spatula presses on the right hand side of the groove in the nucleus and the chopper is pressed on the left hand side of the groove. The two instruments are then moved in opposite directions to create the crack.
3. Two choppers are taken; one introduced through the main incision, the other is introduced through the side port. The two instruments are stabilized at the bottom of the trench and separating the instruments will achieve the crack.

If the nucleus does not crack in these procedures, it is to be understood that the trench is not deep enough. Stop the cracking and fill the anterior chamber with viscoelastics, go in with the Phaco tip and make the trench deeper. Usually it is not necessary to go aggressively to sculpt until you break the posterior capsule. Be gentle in sculpting deeper and try to crack it again. In case of very hard nucleus, it may be difficult to go any deep to achieve the crack, resort to other procedures of nucleus emulsification instead of endangering the posterior capsule or the zonules.

## EMULSIFICATION OF THE HEMI NUCLEUS

Once the nucleus is cracked, the phaco tip is rotated sideways and one half of the nucleus is held in the lower part of the cracked nucleus by introducing the tip using phaco power and held by vacuum at foot position 2 keep a slight pull towards the center and the half nucleus will dislodge and come forward to the central space, now emulsify this by steadying the piece to the phaco tip using the second instrument.

This process of removal of the nucleus is ideal for Grade 2 or 3 Nucleus.

## FOUR QUADRANT DIVIDE AND CONQUER TECHNIQUE

Four Quadrant divide and conquer technique is a commonly used method of nucleus removal for moderately hard nucleus.

After CCC and Hydro procedures, the eye is filled with viscoelastics, the phaco hand piece is taken and tip introduced into the anterior chamber.

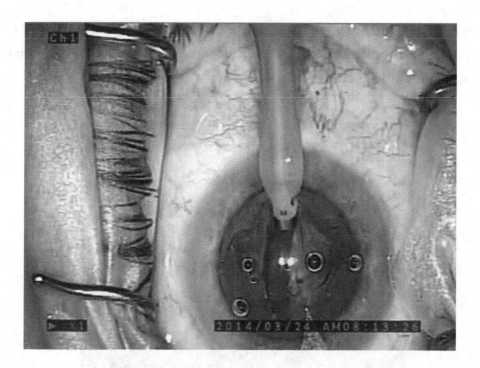

(Fig 24. Creating the trench: Note that the depth of the trench is judged by the texture of the nucleus. Initially the nucleus is very rough and as you go deeper, the Nuclear fibers become smooth and the red reflex is visible.)

**Creating the Trench :**

A trench is made from central position to 6 O clock position as in divide and conquer method. The nucleus is rotated 90 degrees and another trench is made from center up to 6 o clock.

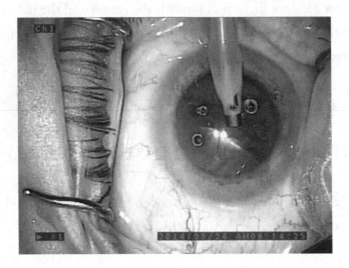

(Fig. 25 Second trench)

The nucleus is rotated another 90 degrees and the first trench is competed from 12 O clock to 6 O clock position. The nucleus is further rotated another 90 degrees and the second trench is completed and thus a cross is created.

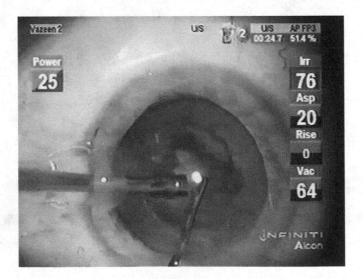

(Fig 26. Four Quadrant technique: Note the cross shape of the two trenches which will break the nucleus in four quadrants.)

Every time the trench is sculpted, it should be three phaco tip deep at the center and two phaco tip wide. One important point is to learn how deep trench is to be made. A rule of the thumb is that the trench should be deep enough so that granular red reflex should be visible through the floor of the trench. This is very gross understatement because; many times the red reflex is not visible due to many other factors. Only experience can tell you how deep the trench should made be to achieve a crack.

**Cracking the Nucleus:**

After the grooves are made, the phaco tip is placed in the depth of the groove with no suction, foot paddle in position 1 to keep the irrigation on and to keep the anterior chamber formed.

A Long 1.5 mm Chopper is taken and introduced through the side port and placed at the depth of the groove next to the phaco tip. Sideways movement of the two instruments will crack the nucleus. This will initiate the crack and continue the crack until the whole nucleus is divided into two halves. The separation has to be complete and strands of cortical fibers clinging to the bottom of the nucleus have to be divided.

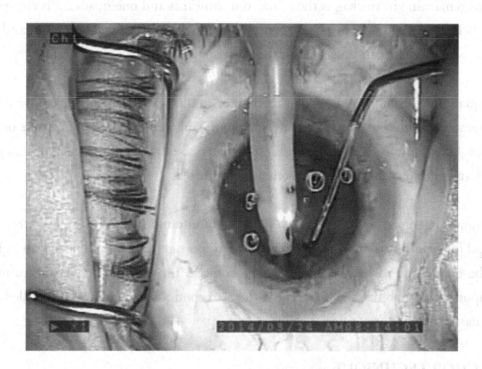

(Fig. 27 Cracking the nucleus : Note the position of the
phaco tip and the Chopper for easy cracking)

Next the nucleus is rotated 90 degrees using the chopper and in the same manner, another crack is made to separate the nucleus into four quadrants by rotating it and continue to crack it and the four quadrants thus made are completely separated.

One point of caution which is often overlooked, the quadrants made in this way are like cake pie pieces cut into four pieces. The pieces are triangular in shape and tip of the quadrant is sharp. Tilting the quadrant tip downwards, may cause damage to the posterior capsule and break it.

## Emulsification of the quadrants:

Emulsification and removal of the quadrants require changing the machine parameters to higher vacuum and less ultrasound power. The phaco tip is directed towards one quadrant, a chopper or a spatula is introduced through the side port and the quadrant is tilted upwards. The phaco tip is engaged and the quadrant is held using vacuum. Phaco power is then used to emulsify and remove the quadrant. Once the first quadrant has been removed, the nucleus is rotated to bring another quadrant to the phaco tip and this is tilted and emulsified as the first one. The half of the nucleus remaining in the bag is then rotated downwards and one quadrant is engaged to be removed. While removing the last quadrant, care is to be taken so that turbulence and surge is minimum, both of these can cause tear of the posterior capsule.

The four quadrant technique is a popular method of emulsification of the nucleus because of its safety to remove the nucleus slowly and safely without danger to the posterior capsule or stress to the zonules. Use of ultrasound energy is also modulated so that minimum energy is spent in the anterior chamber and corneal complications are minimized.

The quadrants are engaged with the phaco tip using ultrasound and pulled slightly to the center of the pupil for emulsification in the iris plane. It is important to place the phaco tip right at the apex of the quadrant and the piece will usually come to the tip directly without tumbling. It is also important to stabilize the quadrant with the second instrument and not pulled into the anterior chamber to perform anterior chamber phaco.

## PHACO CHOP TECHNIQUE

The Phaco chop technique was first described by DR. Kunihiro Nagahara, MD at the 1993 American Society of Cataract and Refractive Surgery (ASCRS) meeting. While the nucleus is impaled and immobilized with the phaco tip, a "chopper" the second instrument is engaged in the equator of the nucleus and chops it toward the phaco tip. The human lens fibers are arranged like the grains of wood and therefore can be cracked with little force.

Woodcutters place a log of wood on a chopping block, and then use an axe to introduce into the log and make a lateral movement of the axe and the log is divided into two pieces.

In this technique, Phaco tip buried into the lens is the Chopping block, Cataract is the Log, and Chopper is used as an Axe to divide the nucleus.

Dr. Nagahara used the same analogy to chop the nucleus into small bite size pieces. Since the introduction of the technique, all phaco surgeons use one or the other modification of the chopping technique for nucleus fragmentation and emulsification.

In the divide and conquer technique and in Four quadrant technique, a tremendous amount of ultrasonic energy is required to make the grooves which are necessary for breaking and separating the quadrants for subsequent emulsification.

The most efficient technique of nucleus disassembly is a purely mechanical one where the nucleus can be chopped and broken into segments. These smaller segments can then easily be removed with relatively little phaco energy.

The basic concept of chopping is holding the nucleus with the phaco tip while the chopping instrument (Chopper) splits it into pieces.

High vacuum level is required to achieve the holding power of the nucleus. The vacuum level should be between 250 mm Hg and 400 mm Hg in peristaltic fluid pump. Total occlusion of the phaco tip is required to achieve the maximum preset vacuum level for a firm hold on the nucleus. First you need to bury the phaco tip into the nucleus using full phaco power (foot position 3). When full occlusion of the Tip is achieved, the vacuum will rise to the preset level then come back to into position 2, of the foot paddle so that the nucleus is now being held by the high vacuum and completely impaled and is ready for chopping.

There are two types of Chopper: 1. Nagahara Type Blunt Chopper or Lieberman microfinger type blunt chopper. 2) Maloney Quick Chopper with sharp tip.

**Horizontal Chopping**: Insertion of the chopper into the anterior chamber is important with the left non dominant hand. Hold the chopper with its tip horizontal, introduce through the side port with the tip horizontal. Then pass the chopper tip under the anterior capsular rim under the epinuclear shell to the equator of the nucleus opposite the site of the Phaco tip, usually at the 5 or 6 O clock positions without damaging the anterior capsule. Once the equator of the nucleus is reached, the two instruments; Chopper and the Phaco tip are compressed. The chopper is pulled towards the phaco tip and, upon contact; the two instruments are moved slightly apart. For most surgeons, this means bringing the chopper towards the left, while the phaco tip is pushed towards the right.

Initial chop cuts through the nucleus distal to the phaco tip. The separating motion continues the fracture along a natural cleavage plane through the proximal remainder of the nucleus. A complete separation of the two pieces is essential for further chopping action to take place. Manual force is used instead of Phaco energy to crack the nucleus.

The nucleus is rotated 30° to 45° clockwise, and the central core of the opposite hemi -nucleus is impaled with the phaco tip in the same manner. A small pie-shaped wedge is now created by the second chop.

Further chopping actions are carried out by rotating the nucleus and it may be divided into 4 to 6 pieces. Removal of the pieces is the next important step.

This first piece is the most difficult to remove. The strong holding force produced by high vacuum of the phaco machine will usually allow elevation of this first piece out of the bag and emulsified while the piece is held steady with the chopper. Alternatively, the curved tip of the chopper can slip behind the equator of this nuclear piece in order to manually tumble it forward into the anterior chamber. This is usually very difficult because, the chopped pieces falls back and fit the other pieces like that of a jigsaw puzzle. To me, holding and pulling the piece out of the bag to a more central position is easier.

The nucleus is rotated further, and the next piece is chopped and removed.

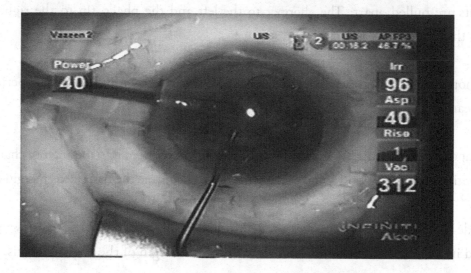

(Fig.28 Chopping the nucleus: Note the position of the chopper and the phaco tip)

**Vertical Chopping**:

Vertical chopping was described by Dr. Hideharu Fukasaku of Japan, and Dr. Abhay Vasavada of India.

In horizontal chopping, the Nagahara-style chopper moves from the periphery toward the phaco tip and this method is partially a blind procedure.

In vertical chopping, first the phaco tip is buried into the nucleus using phaco energy and held at high vacuum. Next, a sharp chopper is used like a spike from above to enter downward into the nucleus just anterior to the centrally buried phaco tip. The most important step is to bury the phaco tip as deeply into the endonucleus as possible. If done correctly, one should actually be able to lift the impaled nucleus upward toward the cornea. Once the fracture begins to propagate, a slight sideways separation of the two instrument tips in opposite direction extends the fracture deeper until the entire nucleus is cleaved in half.

If the nucleus is denser, vertical chopping is a very effective and safe technique. The phaco tip is embedded into the nucleus and the high vacuum level is used to hold the nucleus as before. The sharp tip of the chopper is then placed vertically, into the center of the nucleus, within the margin of the Capsulorhexis.

Once the chopper and phaco tip are both fully buried in the center of the nucleus, the two instruments are pulled apart: The chopper to the left and the phaco tip to the right, thereby separating the two nuclear halves.

Further chopping of the nuclear halves into smaller pieces and emulsification is performed as described earlier.

It is very important to note that, the sharp chopper has to be introduced into the anterior chamber with extreme caution with the tip horizontal because the tip may damage the Iris, rhexis margin or cornea.

Once inside the anterior chamber, it is rotated to bring the sharp tip vertically downward and introduced into the substance of the nucleus, within the margin of the Capsulorhexis.

After the introduction of phaco chop technique, now most of the surgeons use phaco chop in one or the other form, because this reduces the surgical complications and phaco time. The major problem faced during the Nagahara Chopping procedure is the removal of the Copped fragments. The chopped fragments drops back into the capsular bag and fit each other. The pieces have to be pulled out of the bag into the center and freed using vacuum and then emulsified.

## TILT AND CHOP

This is particularly helpful in cases of pseudo exfoliation and where there is zonular weakness.

After Capsulorhexis, hydrodissection and hydrodelineation is performed to delineate and make the size of the nucleus small. The nucleus is tilted and partially prolapsed out of the capsular bag using the second instrument. It is very easy to place the chopper around the lens equator when the nucleus is tilted. The chopper is brought towards the phaco tip and the two instruments are pulled apart to create the two nuclear halves. Further chopping actions are undertaken without putting stress on the zonules by tilting and prolapsing the nucleus out of the bag.

## STOP AND CHOP TECHNIQUE

Phaco Chop technique created a revolution in Phaco surgery; it reduces the time required for phacoemulsification, reduces the phaco energy utilized to emulsify the nucleus and also makes the surgery safer.

The major difficulty in Nagahara Chopping procedure is that, after the nucleus is broken down into several pieces, the pieces fits each other and sits inside the bag as parts of a jigsaw puzzle. Since there is no space in the nucleus to engage and bring the fragments out, it is difficult to hold the pieces and emulsify them. The fact is that the pieces are immobile inside the bag thereby making it difficult to emulsify them. However, once the first piece is brought out of the bag and emulsified, subsequent chopping actions become easier. Dr. Paul Koch MD recognized this problem and in 1994 described the Stop and Chop technique. The technique starts with creating a working space within the nucleus.

Dr. Paul Koch's Stop and Shop Technique starts with creating a central trench and the nucleus is cracked into two pieces and the procedure stops. The chopping action then starts and hence the name "Stop and Chop".

Entry incision is Clear Corneal or Sclero-corneal tunnel, a 5 to 5.5 mm round Capsulorhexis is made and hydrodissection and hydrodelineation is performed, nucleus is tested for rotation.

A trench is made as in divide and conquer technique, the phaco tip is introduced and a groove is created from center to 6 O clock position the nucleus is rotated 180 degrees and the groove is completed from 12 O' clock to 6 O' clock position and the posterior plate is shaved using the red reflex as a guide. Thus a vertical groove from 12 to 6 o clock position is created.

## CRACKING

Once the trench is created and completed, there are many ways for the cracking as described earlier. The most favored technique is to use the phaco tip and a chopper to crack the nucleus.

The phaco tip is held against the Right hand side of the trench with Irrigation on Foot paddle position 1 no vacuum or Ultrasound. A long blunt 1.5 mm chopper is introduced through the side port. Both the instruments are placed at the depth of the trench. The two instruments are then moved to opposite directions and the crack is achieved. The two halves of the nucleus are then completely separated in the bag. Care is taken to separate the cortical fibers at the bottom of the trench and the whole procedure must be performed under perfect vision.

## CHOPPING THE NUCLEUS

The next step after cracking is chopping and emulsification of the nucleus. The nucleus is rotated 90 degrees so that one half of the nucleus comes to lie in the inferior part of the bag, the trench is now horizontal. The machine settings are changed to higher vacuum and ultrasound power is reduced. Taking the advantage of the space created in the nucleus, the phaco tip is engaged in the center of the hemi nucleus using Phaco power in foot position 3.

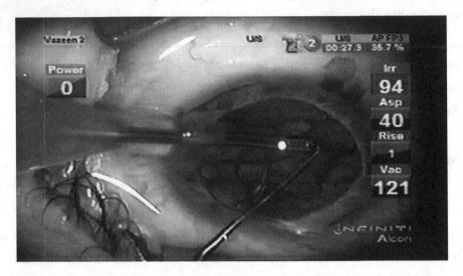

(Fig.29 Chopping and removal of the nucleus : Note that the chopped
nuclear fragments are fed to the phaco tip with the chopper)

The nucleus is held with vacuum and the foot paddle is brought to position 2 and the phaco tip acts as a chopping block. A slight upward pull is maintained in the handpiece. The nucleus half should not be pulled out of the bag which will end up in performing Anterior Chamber Phaco.

The chopper is introduced through the side port and is placed in the peripheral nucleus and introduced inside the nucleus. Chopper is then brought forward toward the phaco tip which remains immobile holding the half of the nucleus. When the instruments approximate each other, they are separated, pushing the chopper to the left and the phaco tip to the right. This is the chopping block analogy described by Nagahara. The phaco tip is the block, the nucleus is the log, and the chopper is the axe. Once the nucleus is broken the quadrant may be further chopped into smaller fragments and emulsified using ultrasound and it may also be possible to emulsify the whole quadrant without further chopping. The nucleus is rotated two clock hours and another piece is chopped and emulsified, this chopping and emulsification is continued until one piece of the nuclear half remains to the left side of the capsular bag. This can be pushed by the chopper toward the phaco tip, engaged, and emulsified easily without any further chopping.

The other half of the nucleus is now free in the bag and this is rotated with the chopper to come to the lower part of the bag. The nucleus is held, immobilized by the phaco tip and chopped in the manner described before and emulsified.

The nucleus can be chopped in 4 to 6 pieces for easy emulsification depending upon the hardness of the nucleus. It is important to have pieces adequately small so they engage at the tip smoothly for emulsification.

## STOP, CHOP AND STUFF TECHNIQUE

After the stop and chop technique was popular, Dr. Avay Vasavada described the technique of Stop Chop and stuff technique which further reduces the use of phaco power. This technique is a modification of stop and chop phacoemulsification.

The CCC, Hydro dissection are performed as usual. The central trench is prepared and the nucleus is cracked in two pieces as described in the stop and chop technique.

When, the chopping is started, chopped fragments are kept small.

The fragments are continuously chopped, and the small pieces are held by vacuum and stuffed inside the phaco tip with the chopper in the non dominant hand. The phaco power is used intermittently for aspiration of the emulsified material and creating the groove. Use of the phaco power to emulsify the fragments is assisted by stuffing the material into the tip by the chopper. This reduces the use of phaco power significantly and is very safe for the cornea especially in hard cataracts.

I love this technique because of the ease of emulsification it produces by stuffing the fragments and also the amount of ultrasound energy in the anterior chamber is reduced significantly. However, this is a bimanual technique and the surgeon has to be very proficient to use both the hands and has to have complete control over the foot paddle

The problem of the technique is, the Phaco tip becomes blunt quickly and needs frequent replacement. Ideally, one phaco tip should be used in each case, but the surgeons in the developing part of the world, tends to reuse the tips several times by autoclaving the tip, but keeping the advantages in mind, replacement of the worn out tip should not be a problem. This is safest method of nucleus removal in small pupil and difficult cases.

**Mechanics of nucleus removal techniques:** Mechanics of every technique of emulsification and removal of the 12 mm nucleus through the 2.8 mm wound requires some understanding.

1) **Mechanics of Chip and Flip Technique:** Chip and flip technique is employed in soft cataracts where it is possible to flip the soft nucleus and remove this by emulsification utilizing short bursts of phaco energy. The mechanics of this technique is the ability of the nucleus to flip over. It is not possible to crack or chop a soft nucleus. Therefore, this is the only safe method for the removal of a soft nucleus. It is not possible to flip a hard nucleus and consequently, this method cannot be applied to a hard nucleus or even a grade 2 or 3 nucleus.

2) **Mechanics of Four Quadrant Divide and Conquer Technique**: The mechanics of Four Quadrant technique is the creation of the trench deep enough so that crack can be achieved. If the trenches prepared are not deep enough, crack cannot be done and consequently the procedure fails. The four quadrants prepared for emulsification must be separated completely and nucleus is mobile for the phaco tip to hold this at the apex of the quadrant and emulsify them one by one. The mechanics is in the mobility of the nucleus and separation of the quadrants. This procedure is extremely safe for cataracts up to grade 3 or moderately hard cataracts. The emulsification is done primarily by the phaco tip and the quadrants can be stabilized by any second instrument like a spatula, chopper or a sinsky hook.

3) **Mechanics of Phaco Chop:** Phaco chop is the most advanced technique in Phacoemulsification. Whatever modality of chopping action is employed, the procedure is partly mechanical partly machine operated. All chopping procedures rely upon the orientation of the Lens Fibers in the cataract. When a groove is created, the nucleus is cut anterior to posterior perpendicular to the orientation of the lens lamellae thus requiring more energy. While chopping is done by immobilizing the nucleus with the phaco tip and then cutting the nucleus mechanically with the chopper parallel to the lens lamellae, thus requiring less energy. Chopping also takes off stress from the zonules and makes it safer in weak zonule cases like mature cataract or pseudo exfoliation cataract. For the phaco tip to cut through the nucleus, the lens must be immobilized. The zonules and capsule grip and fixate the nucleus as the groove is cut by the phaco tip. On the other hand during chopping action, the nucleus is held and immobilized by the phaco tip and works against the force of the chopper, thus reducing the stress on the zonules. All forces are mechanical and

are directed inwards and away from the zonules. The other point in the mechanics of chopping action is placement of the chopper. In horizontal chopping, the chopper must pass below the anterior capsule to brace the equator of the nucleus between epinucleus and the endonucleus. Approximation of the two instruments towards each other yields the necessary force to create the crack and this must be oriented along the lamellae of the nuclear fibers. Perfect visibility of the Capsulorhexis and the depth of the nucleus is a must for this procedure. Vertical chop with a sharp chopper is to be employed with more caution since the sharp tip of the chopper must be kept away from the Capsulorhexis margin and all chopping action must be performed within the Capsulorhexis edge under full visibility. This is an advanced technique and the surgeon must learn and understand the procedure and practice before undertaking and employing chopping action to break the nucleus. Proficient use of the non-dominant hand, movement of the chopper within the anterior chamber, full visibility and learning the mechanics of the cracking action is required before phaco chop is performed. Care is to be taken not to place the chopper outside the anterior capsule on to the zonules and also not to penetrate the rhexis margin by inappropriate maneuver of the chopper. It is also important to break and chop the nucleus into small bite size pieces and it is to be remembered that, the harder the nucleus, the smaller the pieces should be and creating every piece requires separate chopping action to take place. Hold the nucleus firmly utilizing high vacuum, chop to create crack, release, hold again and chop again. Burst mode can be utilized to get a firm purchase of the nucleus. The chopper can be utilized to manually tumble the pie-shaped pieces taking care that this does not somersault forward with its apex hitting the posterior capsule. Understanding the machine settings also plays an important role. Machine settings are to be individualized depending upon the type and capabilities of the machine. During chopping, there are three sequential phaco maneuvers used to remove the nucleus. The first step is the chopping of the nucleus into progressively smaller fragments. In the second step the phaco tip is used to elevate and carry these fragments out of the capsular bag into the pupillary plane. Finally, these pieces are emulsified in the "supracapsular" location at a safe distance from the posterior capsule. For the first two steps, we want our machine to perform Holding action. During emulsification of the nuclear pieces, we need flow ability and controlling the surge. Thus, the machine should be set at high vacuum around 400 mm Hg and this high vacuum increases holding power and prior to phaco chop, a firm purchase of the nucleus is ascertained by complete occlusion of the phaco tip. High vacuum is also required for holding and dislodging the nuclear fragments out of the bag for emulsification. The last step of emulsification produces surge. Therefore, either a machine which has a surge control mechanism is chosen or low vacuum is employed to safely emulsify the fragments. Another useful way to reduce surge is to use a smaller diameter tip which also slow the rate at which emulsification is carried out. Phaco chop is an advanced technique and the surgeon is advised to learn the mechanics and the technique well before utilizing this useful process of removing the nucleus. Almost all phaco surgeons in modern times employ one or the other technique of phaco chop to remove the nucleus.

**SUMMARY: There are many procedures for the removal of the nucleus. However, the new surgeon must pick up, practice and understand the physics behind the particular technique in terms of settings in the particular phaco machine provides to achieve the best surgical outcome. An expert surgeon knows which technique is best with what settings on the machine being used.**

There are basically three types of nucleus in terms of consistency, soft cataract, firm cataract and hard cataract. They differ in their physical properties or behavior during phaco surgery and the settings for a soft cataract will not work for a firm cataract. Therefore, the surgeon must be familiar with the machine and understand the capabilities of the machine at the particular settings. One common mistake is to use the same parameters of settings for the soft and hard cataracts which will run into trouble with one or the other type of cataract. Therefore, there is a need to change the parameters of the machine for every type of cataract and at every step of the surgery. It is a good idea to practice and understand the physical properties of a firm nucleus and the parameters that allow you to remove that nucleus without any complications. Then understand the physical properties of a soft nucleus and understand what parameters are the best to remove that nucleus. You really need to change the technique and the machine parameters based on what the patient is presenting to you. This is what an expert surgeon does over time not to use the same technique for all nucleuses. Therefore, the new surgeon should learn divide and conquer technique on a firm nucleus and then learn chip and flip technique on a soft nucleus and learn the machine parameters for that particular machine what is being used to deliver optimum results without any complications.

## REFERENCES

1.  Pirazzoli G, D'Eliseo D, Ziosi M, Acciarri R. Effects of phacoemulsification time on the corneal endothelium using phacofracture and phaco chop techniques. J Cataract Refract Surg. 1996;22:967-969.

2.  Koch PS, Katzen LE. Stop and chop phacoemulsification. J Cataract Refract Surg. 1994;20:566-570.

3.  Vasavada AR, Desai JP. Stop, chop, chop, and stuff. J Cataract Refract Surg. 1996;22:526-529.

4. Gimbel HV. Divide and conquer nucleofractis phacoemulsification: development and variations. J Cataract Refract Surg. 1991;17:281-291.

5. Shepherd JR. In situ fracture. J Cataract Refract Surg. 1990;16:436-440.

6. Ram J, Wesendahl TA, Auffarth GU, Apple DJ. Evaluation of in situ fracture versus phaco chop techniques. J Cataract Refract Surg. 1998;24:1464-1468.

7. DeBry P, Olson RJ, Crandall AS. Comparison of energy required for phaco-chop and divide and conquer phacoemulsification. J Cataract Refract Surg. 1998;24:689-692.

8. Vasavada A, Singh R, Desai JP. Phacoemulsification of white mature cataracts. J Cataract Refract Surg. 1998;24:270-277.

9. Vasavada A, Singh R. Step-by-step chop in situ and separation of very dense cataracts. J Cataract Refract Surg. 1998;24:156-159.

10. Osher RH, Cionni RJ, Gimbel HV, et al. Cataract surgery in patients with pseudoexfoliation syndrome. Eur J Implant Ref Surg. 1993;5:46-50.

11. Lumme P, Laatikainen LT. Risk factors for intraoperative and early postoperative complications in extracapsular cataract surgery. Eur J Ophthalmol. 1994;4:151-158.

12. I H Fine : The Chip and Flip Phacoemulsification technique Journal of Cataract and Refractive Surgery Issue 3 May 1991; 17(3):366-71.

# Chapter 13
# IRRIGATION AND ASPIRATION

After the nucleus is emulsified and removed, what is left behind is either an epinuclear shell and the entire cortex or just the cortex when the epinucleus is removed along with the nucleus.

If the epinuclear shell is present, the material is thicker and the epinucleus may need to be removed by the phaco hand piece. Under higher vacuum, hold the epinucleus and pull it to the center before removing this with low intermittent phaco power, by momentarily depressing the footplate, if possible flip the whole epinuclear shell which will facilitate removal of the full epinucleus with suction and little ultrasound. The ease of the removal of the epinucleus and cortex will depend on how efficiently the Hydrodissection was performed.

For a beginning surgeon, if the Epinucleus is not easily accessible to the phaco tip, they should stop doing phaco irrespective of the amount of Epinucleus and Cortex left behind. This should be removed by the Irrigation and Aspiration by the I/A handpiece and going slower. The subincisional area is removed first and then sequentially other areas should be cleared by going either at a clockwise or anti clockwise direction.

If the Cortex is found to be attached to the capsule at this stage, the hydrodissection cannula may be used to send jets of BSS to loosen up the cortico capsular adhesions and make the shell more freely mobile.

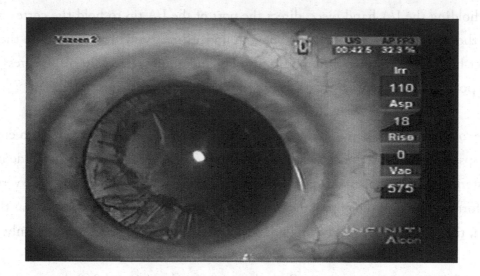

(Fig.30 Cortex after removal of the Nucleus: Note the epinuclear bowl with the cortex)

**Irrigation and Aspiration of Cortex:**

Aspiration and removal of all the cortical mater is very important to reduce and prevent posterior capsular opacification. The posterior capsule is a thin transparent membrane and all the cortical mater must be removed without injury or damage to the posterior capsule. The following points are important while carrying out this task:

1. The cortex or any part of the cortex cannot be removed by the Phaco Handpiece. Therefore, a change from phaco handpiece to Irrigation and Aspiration handpiece is to be made by the assistant.

2. Several port sizes of the I/A tip are available the use of which depends upon the thickness of the remaining cortex. Thus, 0.3, 0.5 and 0.7 mm tips are generally available. A 0.3 mm tip is commonly used.

3. Care must be taken while inserting the I/A tip to the anterior chamber by keeping the Irrigation On with foot plate position at 1 with no aspiration working.

4. The port must always be facing the surgeon or in perfect visibility under the microscope. Slight rotation of the port to face the posterior capsule may engage and damage the Posterior Capsule.

5. While holding the I/A hand piece, direct the port of the I/A tip to hold the cortex and strip it toward the center with the port facing you and under direct visualization remove the cortical strip under high vacuum often 300 to 400 mm Hg and a flow rate of 30 ml. Depress the foot paddle to position 2 and remove the wedge of the cortex after stripping.

6. All the cortical mater is removed by using the same technique. It is dangerous to engage the anterior capsule or the posterior capsule at this vacuum. Therefore most frequent accidental break of the posterior capsule happen during this step of the surgery. The surgeon has to be very careful while performing I/A and the port of the I/A tip must be visible at all times. As soon as the cortex is stripped, the foot paddle must be brought to position 1 with irrigation running only.

7. Striping of the cortex is started at 6 O clock position and continued 360 degrees in steps of 1 to 2 clock hours each time. Once the cortex is engaged in the aspiration tip, further aspiration is stopped and the wage of cortex is brought to the center by slight pull at the hand piece toward the center of the pupil before aspirating this using the preset vacuum.

8. Approach to the subincisional area is most difficult. Some surgeons prefer to aspirate this region first; others tend to go to this area last. Whatever may be the approach, care is to be taken to remove all the cortical mater from subincisional area.

9. The fundamental principle of cortical removal is aspiration. Whether using the Irrigation and Aspiration handpiece or by using the Simco Cannula. There is no harm or shame to use the long time tested simco cannula for aspiration of the cortex for the beginner surgeons if he is more proficient in using this or if the I/A handpiece is not available.

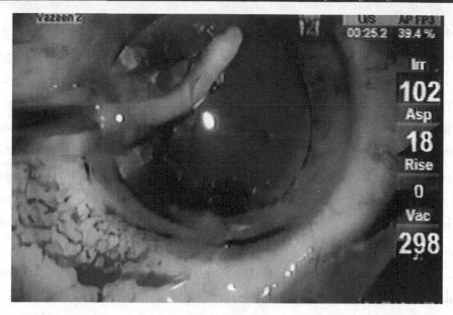

(Fig.31. Irrigation and Aspiration: Note that, it is easier to start the I/A
at the subincisional area first and then going for other regions)

## REMOVAL OF THE SUBINCISIONAL CORTEX:

This is more difficult to approach the area below the main incision for I/A and there are several ways to remove the cortex from the subincisional area. It is better to remove the cortex from the sub-incisional area first and then proceed for the rest of the cortex. The following are some suggestions:

1. **Iris massage:** The cortex at 12 o clock position may be loosened by massaging over the iris with the I/A tip. When the loose cortex shows in the pupillary area, this is aspirated. This procedure may damage the iris or the endothelium and may cause contraction of the pupil.

2. **Irrigation with a J shaped curved cannula :**
   Fit a J shaped irrigating cannula on a 3 cc syringe filled with BSS. Look for a region of clear Capsulorhexis margin at about the midpoint of the pupil. Place the tip of the J-cannula under the cortex against the capsule at 12 o clock position and irrigate. The passing wave of fluid will disengage the subincisional cortical fibers from the capsule and release adhesions at the equator, the cortex should be separated from the posterior capsule at this point and it should be much easier to grasp with the port of the I/A hand piece and aspirated.

3. **Aspiration with Alcon Patented Flexible I/A**

   Use of flexible I/A tip which can be rotated to go under the anterior capsule in the sub incisional area. This is a patented I/A hand piece from Alcon. This Alcon patented instrument uses flexible and steerable aspiration tip for aspiration of cortical mater and includes a tip portion, the configuration of which may be remotely altered to access different areas at a surgical site. The aspiration tip includes a flexible portion which includes a spring material which may be configured in a relaxed and pre-curved state. The aspiration tip is combined with a hand piece assembly which can alter the configuration of the aspiration tip. This facilitates removal of the subincisioal cortex as well as cortex from other parts of the bag.

4. **Use J shaped Simco Cannula: Daljit Singh Simco cannula** shaped and bent like J is available which I have used for many years to aspirate the sub incisional cortex. This works like a standard simco cannula with the difference that, it can be introduced through the main incision or the side port and the subincisional area can be directly approached for irrigation and aspiration.

5. **Aspiration after IOL implant:** This is an alternative procedure. If it becomes difficult to remove the subincisional cortex in the procedures described, it is safer to insert the Intraocular Lens in the bag. The superior edge of the IOL is inserted underneath the cortical mater so that the Optic now lies between the posterior capsule and the cortex.

   The tip of the I/A cannula can now be inserted safely on the optic of the lens and pushed up for aspiration of the cortex. The optic is used as a protection so that the posterior capsule is not injured.

7. **Iris Retraction Method:** This is a desperate method to approach this area. An Iris retractor
   is taken in the non dominant hand and introduced through the main incision and the edge of the iris is gently retracted so that the 12 O clock cortex comes under direct view and the remaining cortex is aspirated.

8. **Leave small amount:** If a very small amount of cortical mater is left deep into the equator of the superior part of the bag and cannot be aspirated, it causes no harm and is absorbed Within two weeks..

6. **CAP VAC :** After the aspiration of the cortical mater is done, the posterior capsule may be polished using 0 to 5 vacuum and low flow rate in CAP VAC mode of the machine to clear any residual cortical fibers present on the posterior capsule with care not to poke the posterior capsule which may break easily.

Irrigation and aspiration of the cortical mater is very important step and most mishap of posterior capsule break happens at this stage. Therefore, care has to be taken to perform all maneuvers and practiced many times before performing this important part of the surgical technique.

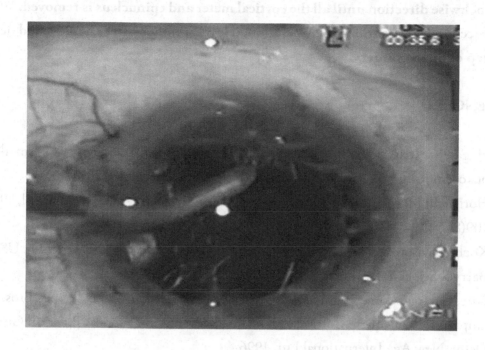

(Fig.32. Irrigation and aspiration of cortex: Note that the cortical fibers are held with vacuum and striped to the center before aspiration.)

## SUMMARY

**The biggest thing to be aware of during this step of surgery is insertion and removal of the Irrigation Aspiration (I/A) tip into the anterior chamber. Most problems with the new surgeons happens as they try to force the tip into the A/C causing Desmet's Detachment and damage to the endothelium or tearing the incision site. Therefore, while entering the A/C slow down the procedure and carefully insert or remove the I/A tip. It is interesting to note that, as you become proficient with Phacoemulsification, most capsular tears seem to happen during I/A. So you need to focus considerably at this step of surgery making sure that the capsular bag is fully formed and posterior capsule is away from the I/A tip at all times. Most surgeons have difficulty with the sub-incisional cortex removal which may result in tear in the posterior capsule or distortion of the corneal wound. If this is happening, stop, and slow down the procedure. Fill up the bag with viscoelastic, insert the IOL in the bag keeping the haptics away from that area and then go in with the I/A tip to aspirate the cortex from the sub incisional area. It comes out lot easier and the IOL is in**

place safely to protect the posterior capsule. It is also safer to start Irrigation and Aspiration of the cortex from the sub incisional area first while there is more cortex present to protect the Posterior capsule and then remove the cortex from other locations going at a clockwise or anticlockwise direction until all the cortical mater and epinucleus is removed. Whatever be the procedure of Irrigation and Aspiration, it is most important to be slow and deliberate at this step of phaco surgery.

## REFERENCES :

1. Hogan JC: Irrigation/Aspiration with changeable tips for cortex removal in small incision phacoemulsification. J Cataract Refract Surg, 1992, Hay; 18(3): 318-20.

2. Horiguchi M: Instrumentation for superior cortex removal. Arch Ophthalmol, 1991, Aug; 109(8): 1170-71.

3. Koch, Davison: Advanced Phacoemulsification Techniques, Slack. Inc. N.J., USA, 1991.

4. Barry S Seibel. Phacodynamics. Slack Inc. N.J., USA 1995.

5. Jaffe, Cataract Surgery and its complications, 4 th Edition, Mosby Jaypee Bros, 1989

6. Gupta VOP. Adequate Cortical Clean Up, Phacoemulsification- A Practical Guide, New Delhi, New Age International Ltd. 1996

7. Boyed Benjamin F. The Modern Mannual Small Incision Extracapsular with Mini –Nuc Technique, Highlights of Ophthalmology, No 1, 2000

## Chapter 14

# INSERTION OF IOL AND REMOVAL OF VISCOELASTIC

Insertion of an IOL in the bag or at the Sulcus is one of the goals of the Intraocular Lens Implant surgery. Usually two types of Lenses are implanted: 1) Rigid PMMA Lens 2) Foldable Intraocular Lens. Anterior chamber lens implantation is rarely performed and has too many complications and therefore discouraged.

**Implantation of Rigid PMMA lenses: (Very rarely performed)**

The PMMA lenses are rare and obsolete now, but the surgeons in developing countries may still need to practice to place PMMA lenses where Foldable lenses are either not available or very costly and patient cannot afford it. Rigid PMMA lenses can not be folded therefore, the incision has to be enlarged up to the diameter of the Optic of the IOL to be implanted. There are different Diameters available, 5.5 mm and 5.1 mm diameter are the most common, but lenses with 6 mm, 6.5 mm or 7 mm diameter are also available. Usually 5.5 mm diameter optic size and 12 mm or, 12.5 mm overall size is optimum for in the bag implantation. Bigger diameter lenses are chosen for implantation in the Sulcus.

The wound is enlarged to 5.5 mm with the appropriate knife with care to keep the corneal tunnel intact. The anterior chamber is filled with Viscoelastics. The lens is held firmly at the Optic – Haptic junction and inserted through the wound under clear visibility. The lower haptic is inserted inside the bag first and the lens is pushed into the anterior chamber with the lower haptic in the bag and the rest of the IOL in the anterior chamber. It is easy to insert the upper haptic in the bag by just holding the upper haptic and by a rotational movement place the haptic inside the upper border of the rhexis margin and release. However, if it is difficult to insert the upper haptic in the bag, the lens has to be dialed in a clockwise direction until the upper haptic goes inside the bag. Filling up the anterior chamber with viscoelastics facilitate this procedure. Keeping one haptic in the bag and the other in the sulcus is not desirable because, this will cause tilting the lens. Keep either both haptic in the bag or dial out and keep both haptics in the sulcus. Placing an IOL in the sulcus will cause 0.5 D refractive change expected postoperatively.

**Implantation of Foldable Intraocular Lenses:**

Several Types of Foldable Intraocular Lenses are available in the market:

1) Single Piece Hydrophobic Acrylic IOL
2) Single piece Hydrophilic Acrylic IOL
3) Multi piece Acrylic IOL
4) Silicon Lenses
5) Other Lenses with surface modifications
6) Speciality IOL

Each of these Intraocular Lenses behaves in a different manner while implanting.

First Step to implant a foldable lens is to load the lens into the Injector. Every IOL company has its own Injector System; each one of them has a different way to load the lens into the injector.

Some companies have Disposable Injectors. Others have cartridge to be loaded and fitted to the injector system. Some companies have preloaded lens in the injector.

In any case the surgeon must learn how to load and unload the foldable lens into the injector and out of it. All companies will supply ample number of practice lenses and injectors to practice.

I have seen many surgeries ruined due to faulty use of the Injector, therefore, practice well both Loading and Unloading before you start to use the particular lens and injector.

After loading the lens in the injector, look at it under the microscope light so that, none of the part of the lens is caught on to the wings of the cartridge.

The anterior chamber is filled with viscoelastic. The tip of the injector is introduced into the tunnel and is advanced to the center of the pupil. Gentle push on the plunger will advance the lens in the injector and the lower haptic will unload which will be visible this is to be placed in the bag first. Advancing the plunger further will deliver the optic and the last to unload is the trailing haptic. Slight push on the optic will usually place the upper haptic in the bag. If this do not happen, dialing the lens to introduce the upper haptic in the bag may be necessary. If the anterior chamber is shallow, placement of the lens in the bag will be difficult. Filling up the anterior chamber with viscoelastic will aid in correct placement of the lens in the bag.

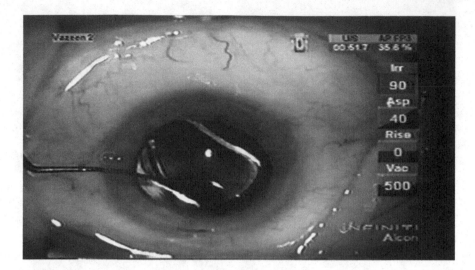

(Fig.33 Insertion of IOL in the bag : Note that the bag must be filled with viscoelastic and the injector is slowly withdrawn as the lens is injected in the bag.)

Sudden push on the plunger may forcefully unload the lens and damage the bag or the capsule.

The injector tip is removed from the anterior chamber slowly and the lens is centered using the dialer.

One point is worth mentioning here, the Hydrophilic lenses unfolds quicker and almost instantaneously unfolds itself to normal position and it is easier to dial it into the bag. If the upper haptic is not in the bag already, refill the anterior chamber with viscoelastic and with the tip of a dialer, press on the optic and the lens will get into the bag easily.

Hydrophobic lenses unfold slowly; sometimes it may take up to two minutes to unfold itself after implantation. The surgeon has to wait for this period of time, which may feel very long during surgery. While the lens is unfolding, just wait and don't dial or don't try to force it unfold. Once unfolded, the lens can then be dialed in the bag to center it properly.

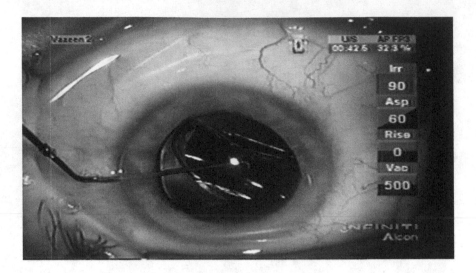

(Fig. 34 Unfolding of IOL after implantation in the Bag :
Hydrophobic lenses take longer to unfold)

When we started to learn Phaco surgery, the injector system was more complicated to handle. Now the new injector systems are much better and in the future new designs of lenses and injectors will come with preloaded lens in the injector. Some injectors may have a wing which may cause the edge of the capsulorhexis margin to be caught and cause damage of the bag and thus a good surgery may be spoiled. Some injectors may need special technique to load the lens and while loading, the haptics of the IOL may be captured by the wings and the IOL may be torn during delivery. Removal of the IOL from the anterior chamber is not easy and re insertion of a new IOL becomes necessary. Therefore, the surgeon must be vigilant so that these unwanted complications do not happen.

## SUMMARY OF LENS INSERTION

Care is necessary at this step of surgery to avoid unnecessary complications. The point to note is, as you insert the lens; slowly remove the injector from the eye. This will allow the necessary space required for the lens to unfold. Initially you may have put the injector 2 to 3 mm inside the anterior chamber, as you push the plunger, the lens starts to come out of the tip and at the same time you should slowly start to come out of the anterior chamber. This movement allows the inferior haptic of the lens to enter the capsular bag smoothly. The upper haptic also goes into the bag if the anterior chamber is well formed. This gives us the best chance of insertion and centering of the Intraocular Lens without causing complications.

## VISCOELASTIC REMOVAL

The last step in Phaco surgery is to remove the viscoelastic, using the I/A handpiece from the anterior chamber. This can be done with a Simco cannula too if I/A handpiece is not available.

Introduce the I/A cannula into the anterior chamber and press the foot paddle to start I/A to begin aspiration of the viscoelastic. Don't rush to remove the viscoelastic, remove slowly and as much as possible.

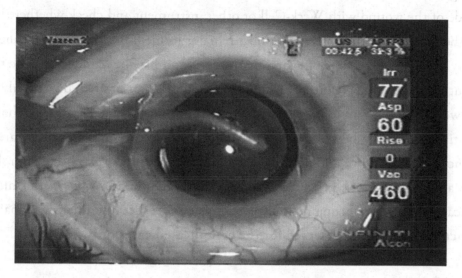

(Fig. 35 Removal of Viscoelastic : This should be as complete
as possible with slow movement of the I/A tip)

Some surgeons are very aggressive to remove the viscoelastic from the anterior chamber, from behind the optic and the corners of the anterior chamber. While this is good to remove all the viscoelastics, but some viscoelastic is always left behind in the anterior chamber which will go out of the anterior chamber in a couple of hours. My advice is not to be too aggressive endangering the posterior capsule but try to remove as much as possible taking time to do the Irrigation and aspiration.

It is to be remembered that, viscoelastics are thick substances and require meticulous aspiration in order to remove this completely.

Small amount of viscoelastic left behind the IOL will be absorbed in 24 hours time, if in doubt, give one tab. Acetazolamide on discharge and one on the first postoperative day. Slight spike of increased IOP will happen while the viscoelastic is being absorbed but this usually settles down quickly.(Irrigation and Aspiration of Viscoelastic)

## Wound closure

Next thing is to test the wound for any leaks. A 2 cc syringe is taken filled with BSS and a Cannula is fitted. Hydrate the lips of the cornea to seal the wound well. Check if there is any leak by irrigating the anterior chamber with BSS through the side port. Press on the eye ball on the opposite side of the wound with Weck-Cell or other instrument and check whether there is any leak from the wound and the anterior chamber remains formed. If it happens that the wound is not properly water sealed in spite of hydrating the cornea, it may be required to close the wound with one suture with 10/O Nylon. Suturing of the wound is not desired, but it is always better to seal the wound rather than to keep an open leaking wound to get a flat anterior chamber next day. This stitch can easily be removed after two weeks. Topical antibiotic drops are instilled. Sub-conjunctival injection of antibiotics may be given if the surgery has become prolonged for any reason and the surgery is performed under regional anesthesia. While performing surgery under topical anesthesia, subconjunctival injection is avoided because this is very painful. **Any subconjunctival injection is reserved for the complicated cases only.**

## REFERENCES:

1.  Martin RG, Sander DR et al.: Effect of posterior chamber intraocular lens design and surgical placement on postoperative outcome. J Cataract Refract Surg. 1992 July, 18(4): 33-41.
2.  Brint SF. Ostrick-M: The evolution of small incison cataract surgery with foldable lOLs. J Am Optom Assoc. 1992 May; 62(5); 365-71
3.  Martin RG, Sander DR et al.: Effect of posterior chamber intraocular lens design and surgical placement on postoperative outcome. J Cataract Refract Surg. 1992 July, 18(4): 33-41.
4.  Nishi ONishi KSakanishi K Inhibition of migrating lens epithelial cells at the capsular bend created by the rectangular optic edge of a posterior chamber intraocular lens. Ophthalmic Surg Lasers. 1998;29587- 594
5.  Masket Sed Consultation section: cataract surgical problem. J Cataract Refract Surg. 1998;241554- 1561
6.  Holladay JTAng APortney V Analysis of edge glare phenomena in intraocular lens edge designs. J Cataract Refract Surg. 1999;25748- 752

7.  Landry RA Unwanted optical effects caused by intraocular lens positioning holes. J Cataract Refract Surg. 1987;13421- 423

8.  Shah SMSpalton DJ Changes in anterior chamber flare and cells following cataract surgery. Br J Ophthalmol. 1994;7891- 94

9.  Amon MMenapace R In vivo documentation of cellular reactions on lens surfaces for assessing biocompatibility of different intraocular lens implants. Eye. 1994;8649- 656

10. Pande MUrsell PSpalton DJ Postoperative inflammatory response to phacoemulsification and extracapsular cataract surgery: aqueous flare and cells. J Cataract Refract Surg. 1996;22770- 774

11. Oshika TTsuboi SYaguchi S et al. Comparative study of intraocular lens implantation through 3.2- and 5.5-mm incisions. Ophthalmology. 1994;1011183- 1190

12. Ohara K Biomicroscopy of surface deposits resembling foreign-body epithelioid cells on implanted intraocular lenses. Am J Ophthalmol. 1985;99304- 311

13. Nichamin LD Astigmatism control. Ophthalmol Clin North Am 2006;19 (4) 485- 493

14. Leffler CTJavey GMahmood MA Prediction of postoperative astigmatism in cataract surgery. Can J Ophthalmol 2008;43 (5) 551- 554

15. Covert DJHenry CRKoenig SB Intraocular lens power selection in the second eye of patients undergoing bilateral, sequential cataract extraction. Ophthalmology 2010;117 (1) 49- 54

16. Oshima YTsujikawa KOh AHarino S Comparative study of intraocular lens implantation through 3.0 mm temporal clear corneal and superior scleral tunnel self-sealing incisions. J Cataract Refract Surg. 1977; 23 (3): 347-353.

# Chapter 15

# PRECAUTIONS AND DIFFICULTIES IN PHACO SURGERY

During Phaco surgery and cataract surgery in general, all the steps has to be accurate and as planned. If one step goes wrong, all other steps will become difficult and may proceed to irreparable damage.

Therefore, the surgeon must be able to anticipate the complications during surgery and have full knowledge to handle the difficult situations, correct them instantly and efficiently. Right from the incision to Lens implantation and ending the procedure, all the steps are arranged as pearls on a string. If one pearl is displaced, the whole chain falls apart.

One point I would like to mention here is that, no matter what procedure you adopt to perform the surgery, 2.5 mm incision or a 6 mm incision, phaco or no phaco, stitch or no stitch, the end result is important. If the vision can be restored as expected at the end of the post operative period, be it one day or six weeks will not matter much except needing reassurance. But if the problem goes out of hand which lead to complications, that are more difficult to handle or are irreparable, and the vision can not be restored as expected, this becomes distressing to the patient and cause disappointment. The patient wants good visual outcome irrespective of the length of the recovery period.

**For the beginning surgeon it is a very good idea to be familiar with the steps of phaco surgery and device a plan for the possibility of each of the steps going wrong and when it happens in real time, you can refer to your devised plan and act accordingly. This is like a Golfer who practices to take shots from behind a rock and when it happens in real time, he stays calm and knows exactly what to do.**

If you run into difficulties during surgery, tackle the situation so that the end result is satisfactory. Don't panic if things do not go as planned, rectify the problem and proceed as required and you will have nothing to regret. The corrective steps for some of the problems are discussed in this chapter, and I must say that these are only suggestions at the presented situation and are to be considered as reflection of our experiences. Other surgeons may tackle the situation by a different approach depending upon their personal practical experience.

## DIFFICULTY IN INCISION

Entry to the anterior chamber requires an incision and is a very important step in phacoemulsification. Self sealing valve incision through a Scleral tunnel or through a corneal tunnel is the two procedures of entry to the Anterior Chamber.

However, when premature direct entry to the anterior chamber happens due to any reason where the corneal valve is not created, phaco surgery is impossible through this incision. If phaco surgery is tried, this will lead to iris prolapse through the incision, when prolapsed iris is reposted, pupil constricts becomes small which is difficult to dilate, subsequent reentry with the phaco probe causes further constriction of the pupil, iris damage and steps go on to be difficult.

For example, in a similar situation, if a corneal tunnel entry was made but the knife entered the eye due to the use of sharp knife at a wrong plane and the anterior chamber is entered directly without creating a corneal valve, best suggestion is to close this incision using one 10/0 Nylon suture and a second corneal tunnel is made two clock hours away from the first incision, this will require adjustment of the sitting position of the surgeon and adjustment of the microscope. The surgery is performed through the second incision and the new side port usually with no difficulty. Check for wound integrity at the end of the surgery. The second incision will be self sealing. The suture of the first incision is kept for about four to six weeks and can be removed. The end surgical result will have no reflection of the problem encountered.

If the surgery was started with a Scleral Tunnel at 12 O clock position and the anterior chamber was entered directly without constructing a corneal valve, take a pause in surgery and examine the hardness of the cataract under the microscope. If you think that the nucleus is not so hard and can be emulsified easily, then close the first incisions with one to three interrupted 10/O Nylon sutures and proceed with a temporal corneal tunnel and complete the surgery through the second incision. If you think that the nucleus is hard and phaco will be difficult, then enlarge the sclera- corneal incision to 6 mm and convert to SICS and at the end of the SICS surgery check the wound which usually requires one to three scleral sutures to secure the wound because no corneal tunnel was constructed.

Remember that, direct entry incisions where corneal valve is absent, or a short corneal tunnel is constructed, always require sutures to seal the wound which can be removed after four to six weeks.

The point of all these is to create a game plan before it goes wrong and not trying to figure out what to do in real time surgery. If you panic at any point more mistakes will be made and the surgery will be more difficult. I want to point out that, a good surgeon get great results after a good surgery and an excellent surgeon get good results when there are complications. Every surgeon will have his or her share of the complications in the clinical life.

## DIFFICULTY IN CAPSULORHEXIS:

Performing a continuous circular Capsulorhexis CCC is a commitment for phaco surgery. If you fail to make a capsulotomy in which the margin is continuous, the commitment is broken and conversion to SICS may be necessary. For now, I shall discuss what needs to be done if Capsulorhexis goes wrong.

**Difficult situation 1**: Suppose you have introduced the cystitome and started rhexis, but instead of a Puncture, you get a vertical or horizontal slit and it is difficult to raise the flap to initiate the tear, stop and make the cystitome tip horizontal come out of the anterior chamber. Inject good viscoelastic like Healon, enlarge the incision to 2.5 mm and introduce an angled vannas scissor and make a small cut at one of the margins of the slit and start the rhexis with forceps, when completing the tear, slightly overrun the original cut to make the rhexis margin continuous. Round or oval is not a prerequisite, continuous rhexis margin is important.

**Difficult situation 2** : Suppose you have started Capsulorhexis and is going smoothly, but coming to 6'O clock position, it starts to run away and this can happen at any clock hour position. Stop the rhexis immediately and bring the cystitome out of the A/C. The main reason of rhexis run away or misdirection is fall of positive pressure in the Anterior Chamber. Fill up the A/C with viscoelastic and start the rhexis from the opposite direction in opposite clock hours, from the other end of the cut. If you had been doing anticlockwise rhexis, now you have to go in clockwise direction and vice versa. This may be difficult to raise the flap in the opposite direction, try it with the forceps but if you fail to initiate the tear, don't spoil the margin, get in with an angled vannas scissors and make a cut in the margin to raise the flap. Continue the rhexis in the opposite direction to meet the margin at the first end; try to overrun the margin to create a smooth round edge.

**Difficult situation 3**: If one of the rhexis ends was misdirected and rhexis was started with the second end in the opposite direction as described earlier, but the end of the second flap also starts to run away, stop, don't panic insert viscoelastic and try to redirect the rhexis with forceps again and if this also fails, convert to can opener capsulotomy and cut the tags of the capsule if present with vannas scissors and remove the anterior capsule. In some cataracts, it is difficult to perform a rhexis for example in fibrotic capsule. Can opener capsulotomy is a good option in these cases. Enlarge the incision and convert to SICS. This will give very good post operative results and you can also implant a Foldable Acrylic lens or a PMMA lens. As long as the posterior capsule is intact, you are safe and the surgical result is acceptable whether phacoemulsification or SICS is performed.

**Difficult situation 4:** If during Capsulorhexis, the margin is not visible, stop the procedure and find out where the rhexis margin is. If that is not possible, stain the anterior capsule with Trypan blue and once the margin is visible, start the rhexis again. Rhexis is never a blind procedure and never attempt to perform a rhexis without clear visibility. If the capsulorhexis margin is not visible in spite of these attempts, convert to Can Opener capsulotomy and SICS.

## DIFFICULTIES IN HYDRODISSECTION:

**Difficult situation 1**: Hydrodissection in Posterior Polar cataract is difficult and dangerous. Perform Hydrodelineation in these cases and manage the case as described in the chapter on Posterior Polar Cataract. Slow hydrodissection or hydrodelineation is the key and don't force fluid at any time in these types of cataract.

**Difficult situation 2 :** You have introduced the cannula under the capsule and pushed fluid, but a fluid wave did not propagate. You actually have given a rinse of the outer side of the nucleus. Go in at a different location and advance the tip of the cannula a little further before injecting BSS. If you can see a fluid wave propagating, keep on injecting until the wave is complete.

**Difficult situation 3 :** You have performed hydrodissection but the nucleus do not rotate. There are capsule cortical adhesions. Take a J shaped irrigation cannula, insert the cannula under the anterior capsule at 12 O clock position gently inject some fluid and repeat this in all other quadrants thus trying to separate the adhesions. Remember that, you are no longer performing hydro dissection; you are actually making hydro separation. Therefore a strong jet of fluid is not required. You need a gentle rinse to free the adhesions which is between the anterior capsule and the superficial cortex. If you do not still get rotation, do not attempt to rotate the nucleus forcibly, this will exert stress on the zonules. Always remember to gently press on the nucleus to release and egress fluid out of the nucleus and not let the fluid get trapped inside the nucleus. You can start Phaco by sculpting the nucleus a bit wide and deep trench and crack the nucleus. Further chopping action will free the nucleus from its adhesions. Once you can chop one fragment of the nucleus and emulsify the fragment, the space created will allow the nucleus to rotate and you can usually proceed with phaco surgery and rotation of the nucleus without any further problems.

**Difficult situation 4:** What happens if you fail to get any hydrodissection at all, fluid injected from different positions only returns back and neither produces a fluid wave, or the nucleus lifts up? This is a hard cataract with capsulolenticular adhesions. You shall have to convert to another form of nucleus delivery. Don't try to inject fluid or rotate the nucleus forcibly. There are other better methods of safe nucleus delivery and visco expression will achieve good result and that is what you want.

## DIFFICULTIES IN EMULSIFICATION OF THE NUCLEUS:

Many difficulties are encountered when emulsifying the nucleus. It is important to recognize these difficult situations and tackle them early enough so that major problems can be avoided.

1. **Chip and Flip Technique:**

   In chip and flip method, one problem may arise when the bowl is excavated, but the nucleus does not come forward. Shave the posterior plate and try to break. If you cannot achieve a break in the nuclear rim, you may have done enough phaco and finished the hard part of the nucleus. What is remaining is a bowl of soft epinucleus and cortex. Remember the rest of the bowl of Epinucleus and Cortex is soft. Stop further phaco at this point.

   Take the hydrodissection cannula again insert the cannula just under the anterior capsular rhexis margin and loosen the cortex at different sites. You are not doing hydrodissection now and therefore the force of the fluid does not need to be much, just enough to loosen the cortex from the capsule at the equator.

   Now change the parameters on the phaco machine. Reduce the ultrasound power to 30 and aspiration at 200 mm Hg and flow rate to 25.

Try to hold the remainder of the nucleus in the inferior part by aspiration force only, not by phaco energy. Foot Paddle position 2. Now exert gentle pulling towards the center, break a small fragment of the nucleus using a blunt chopper.

Once a small piece of the nucleus is removed, hold the margin of the broken nucleus, rotate and pull the soft nucleus out of the bag and the nucleus may flip at this point, remove the soft epinucleus shell along with cortex by gentle phaco. Next you may proceed to Irrigation and Aspiration of the cortex using the I/A hand piece.

## 2. Divide and conquer Technique:

It is possible that after making the crater, you have engaged the handpiece and spatula in the lower part of the nucleus but cannot divide it. The reason in this situation is, the trench is not deep enough. Stop the cracking and fill the anterior chamber with viscoelastics, go in with the Phaco tip and make the trench deeper, try not to be aggressive to end up in breaking the posterior capsule. Be gentle in sculpting deeper and try to crack again. In case this attempt is also unsuccessful, then use the next trick.

You can understand that the crater has been made and there is space in the center, the half eaten nucleus, epinucleus and cortical shell is still present in the bag. Take a hydrodissection right angled cannula, insert just under the anterior capsule in multiple places and send gentle jets of fluid to separate the cortex and capsule as much as possible. Change the phaco parameters to higher vacuum.

Now insert the Phaco tip again and approach the 6 O clock or 5 O clock position. Hold the nucleus in the inferior part using vacuum pull the nuclear rim to tilt it slightly. Take a blunt chopper in the left hand and chop a small piece of the nucleus from this position.

Once this is done the rest of the nucleus will become weaker and will collapse due to the crater made. This can be removed using vacuum, tilt and chop and use of intermittent phaco power. Most important thing is clear visibility at all these steps, look at the tip of the instruments that you are using inside the anterior chamber and look at the structures you are holding by them.

3. **Four quadrant Cracking Phaco Technique :**

In four Quadrant technique, the first problem may happen while cracking the quadrants. If they do not break easily, less sculpting has been done and sculpt more using down slopping sculpting procedure, rotate the nucleus and sculpt the second groove also. Now crack can be achieved easily into four quadrants.

Next problem is faced while emulsifying the quadrants. Remember not to hold the nucleus from the top position. Tilt the nucleus quadrant with the second instrument to bring the apex of the quadrant to the phaco tip, then hold and emulsify in the pupillary plane. Another mistake is to pull the quadrant to the anterior chamber to perform anterior chamber phaco and cause corneal damage.

It may happen that, after the quadrants are broken, the first quadrant cannot be brought to the phaco tip. There are cortical adhesions, lift the apex of the piece up with the spatula and hold to emulsify. The Nuclear Quadrants should come to the phaco tip easily. If the pieces do not come to the phaco tip, do not pull on the quadrant forcibly. Release the quadrant, rotate the nucleus, grab the second piece, and third or fourth. One of the quadrants will come easily and naturally to the phaco tip and once if you have emulsified one quadrant, the other quadrants will easily come to the phaco tip.

There are times when the most dangerous problem may happen. If you find that, after cracking and emulsifying one quadrant, the nucleus is no longer rotating and coming to the tip, it may indicate that, the posterior capsule has broken and vitreous is present in the anterior chamber.

The A/C may suddenly become deep. Don't panic; come out of the anterior chamber without further delay keeping the A/C formed. Now enlarge the incision to 5 mm or 5.5 mm, using the sinsky hook or any other hook pull the quadrants to the anterior chamber one by one. The quadrants can then be pulled out using McPherson's forceps. Do not use any pushing action or irrigation to deliver the quadrants that will enlarge the posterior capsular rent if happened and can endanger dropping of the nucleus or nucleus quadrants in to the vitreous cavity.

After the nuclear fragments are brought out of the A/C use the simco cannula irrigation and gentle aspiration to clear as much cortex as possible. If there is vitreous in the anterior chamber, perform anterior vitrectomy and manage as a case of vitreous loss. If the rent is small and the anterior capsulorhexis margin is intact, IOL can be placed in the sulcus after appropriate vitrectomy is performed.

4. **Difficult situations in Phaco Chop:**

In Phaco chop technique, the essence of the procedure is to crack the nucleus in several pieces.

It may so happen that, when we try to chop after burying the tip, crack do not appear. This may be due to the fact that, a small chopper is being used. Change to a 1.5 mm chopper and insert the tip of the chopper up to its bend into the nucleus. It is safe and nothing to be afraid of because, the Nucleus is 2 mm deep at this situation and a crack will definitely start.

It may so happen that, trying to chop and separating the instruments results only insertion of the chopper in the nucleus. This is because the nucleus is soft and not hard enough to chop.

Simply consider other methods of nucleus removal, such as chip and flip method or divide and conquer method.

In very hard Cataract, it is difficult to insert the chopper into the substance of the nucleus. Stop the technique and try Stop and Chop method instead.

The other difficulty may be that even after good chops and nucleus has been divided into several small pieces, the first piece does not come forward for emulsification. Do not exert pull on the fragment; this will result into break of the zonules. The problem here is, the Capsulorhexis is smaller than required. A rhexis of at least 5.5 mm is required in this situation. Stop the technique, use Dye to stain the Capsule and make a bigger rhexis using the angled Vannas scissors and Rhexis forceps. If you can make a bigger rhexis try to remove the pieces. If this does not work and the pieces are still fixed inside the bag like a jigsaw puzzle, it is better to try other procedures like converting to SICS.

## 5. Difficulties in Stop and chop technique:

Stop and chop technique is a very safe method of nucleus removal and requires least amount of ultrasound power necessary to remove the nucleus than any other nucleus disassembly procedures. But the surgeon may confront difficult situations while performing the procedure. Firstly, the groove is difficult to make because the phaco tip do not cut, this may be due to worn out tip or using less power, increase the power settings to 90 change to a new tip and try again.

Secondly, the nucleus do not crack easily, in this case, the groove is not deep enough. Try to sculpt little more to make a deeper groove. The other reason may be that you are using a small chopper. Take a 1.5 mm chopper and position the chopper at the bottom of the trench. After cracking the nucleus, make sure all the strands of the cortex has been separated and two hemi nucleuses are completely separate. When chopping is started, the phaco tip may not hold the nucleus strongly enough for the chopping action. There are two reasons for this, the tip is not buried enough into the nucleus or the sleeve is preventing the tip to enter the nucleus. The sleeve of the phaco tip needs to be adjusted and attempt should be made to bury the tip at the densest part of the nucleus. The second reason is the vacuum of the machine is not high enough to hold the nucleus, increase the vacuum setting of the machine. Anterior chamber Phaco is to be avoided at all times, all chopping and emulsification has to be done at the Iris Plane.

### Difficulties during Irrigation and Aspiration:

Difficulties may arise during irrigation and aspiration and as discussed earlier, posterior capsule complications occur more often at this stage of surgery. First problem, nothing happens after introduction of I/A cannula and pressing on the foot paddle. This may be due to the fact that the port is blocked and the I/A tip needs to be changed which will solve the problem.

The other problem frequently faced during I/A is removal of a small plaque of cortical mater which is lying on the posterior capsule. This happens mostly in Posterior Sub capsular and Posterior Polar Cataracts. Try to hold it with very low vacuum like 10 vac, if you can dislodge it, bring it to the A/C and aspirate it. If you feel it is dangerous to work on the posterior capsule, better leave it alone and implant the IOL. While implanting the optic of the IOL, the cortical mater may dislodge. Even if it does not and you have left it on the posterior capsule, chances are that it will be absorbed in few weeks time.

There may be early posterior capsular opacity and this can be easily removed by YAG LASER three months after surgery. But desperate try to remove it to cause a posterior capsule tear is not worth at all and the post operative result will be worse than if left it alone and perform YAG LASER posterior capsulotomy later.

### Difficulties during insertion of the IOL:

While insertion of an IOL with the injector is a very straight forward step and at the end of the surgery nobody expects to face any difficulty, yet this is a potential step for things to go seriously wrong. Firstly, if the lens is not properly loaded in the injector and the trailing haptic is caught in the injector, forceful attempt of delivery of the lens to the Anterior Chamber may cause delivery of a broken lens into the A/C. Remember, once the lens is out of the injector, it can not be brought out of the anterior chamber through the small 2.8 or 3 mm incision. You have got to enlarge the incision to the size of the optic of the lens you are implanting to remove it, load another IOL in the injector and insert the new IOL. The wound may not be self sealing anymore; one stitch may be required to close the wound. Another problem I have seen is that, on an attempt of forceful injection, the IOL may suddenly come out of the injector and hit the posterior capsule and break it. Insertion of the IOL is a gentle procedure, please do not apply force to inject the IOL and have patience at this step. It is important to keep the anterior chamber formed while implanting the IOL. If the lens is not moving smoothly in the injector, bring the tip of the injector out of the wound, remove the lens from the injector reload again using a new injector or cartridge and inject slowly and smoothly. It is always safer to withdraw the injector slowly as you are injecting the IOL in the bag. This ensures entry of the lens into the bag and proper centering.

### REFERENCES :

1. Osher R, Cionni R. The torn posterior capsule: Its intra-operative behavior, surgical management, and long-term consequences. *J Cataract Refract Surg.* 1990;16:490-494.

2. Powe NR, Schein OD, et al. Synthesis of the literature on visual acuity and complications following cataract extraction with intraocular lens implantation. *Arch Ophthalmol.* 1994;112:239-252.

3. Fishkind WJ. Unexpected vitrectomy as a complication of cataract surgery. *J Cataract Refract Surg.* Best Papers of Session 1994; 54-57.

4.  Gimbel HV. Divide and conquer nucleofractis phacoemulsification: development and variations. *J Cataract Refract Surg.* 1991;17:281-291.

5.  Vasavada AR, Desai JP. Stop, chop, chop, and stuff. *J Cataract Refract Surg.* 1996;22:526-529.

6.  Koch PS, Katzen LE. Stop and chop phacoemulsification. *J Cataract Refract Surg.* 1994;20:566-570.

7.  Vasavada A, Singh R. Step-by-step chop in situ and separation of very dense cataracts. *J Cataract Refract Surg.* 1998;24:156-159.

8.  Melles G, de Waard P, Pameyer J, Beekhuis W. Trypan blue capsule staining to visualize the capsulorhexis in cataract surgery. *J Cataract Refract Surg.* 1999;25:7-9.

9.  Horiguchi M, Miyake K, Ohta I, Ito Y. Staining of the lens capsule for circular continuous capsulorhexis in eyes with white cataract. *Arch Ophthalmol.* 1998;116(4):535-537

# Chapter 16
# INTRAOPERATIVE COMPLICATIONS

Complications can happen during Cataract Surgery and the success of a good surgeon is not only to perform surgery in an ideal situation, but also to be prepared to tackle the surgery if things go wrong at any time and take corrective measures. The mark of a great surgeon is who gets great results in spite of the complications.

The complications described are common during cataract surgery but the list is not inclusive of all the complications that can happen during the procedure. The managements described are based on the personal experience of both the authors and once the basics are learned, the surgeon may manage the complication as he or she feels comfortable.

**Common Surgical Complications:**

1. Damaged corneal tunnel and Wound Leak
2. Desmet's Detachment
3. Rhexis Runaway and Failed Rhexis
4. Constriction of Pupil and Shallow anterior chamber.
5. Intra operative rise of IOP and positive vitreous pressure
6. Break in the Posterior Capsule
7. Nucleus Drop
8. Zonular Dehiscence
9. Suprachoroidal and Expulsive Hemorrhage

## DAMAGE TO THE CORNEAL TUNNEL

Damage to the corneal or Scleral tunnel may happen due to wrong construction of the tunnel or using a blunt knife and utilizing force to enter the anterior chamber. If this happens, the margin of the tunnel may be ragged or there may be premature direct entry to the anterior chamber. In this situation, stop the surgery, introduce Viscoelastic, assess the situation, if the tunnel is damaged to the point where phaco surgery will be difficult because of leakage and iris prolapse, it is better to close the incision with one or two vertical suture and perform the surgery through a second site with a new knife and a new tunnel which has already been described.

**Desmet's Detachment :**

Detachment of the Desmet's membrane is not an uncommon situation. This may be caused by repeated entry to the anterior chamber with the phaco probe or the second instrument or using a blunt knife to create the tunnel. Recognition of the detachment is important and if detected, fill up the anterior chamber with viscoelastic and enter under the detached Desmet's membrane every time you enter the eye. If overlooked, this may cause a big detachment of the Desmet's Membrane may strip off and hang like a curtain, causing failed surgery due to corneal edema.

Small detachments of Desmet's membrane is of no concern, and filling up the anterior chamber (A/C) with BSS at the end of surgery will appose the Desmet's to the corneal stroma and will heal without problem. If the detachment is bigger and do not stay apposed with BSS at the end of surgery, this will need internal Tamponade by air.

In this case, after completion of surgery, fill up the anterior chamber with sterile air to internally Tamponade the Desmet's membrane apposing it to the Stroma. I do not trust operation room ambient air to be sterile. Therefore, to get sterile air, take a sterile 2 cc disposable syringe and pull the plunger out as far as it can go inside the intact plastic package, then open the package and introduce the air inside the syringe with a freshly opened cannula into the anterior chamber. There are other ways to get sterile air but ambient air in the operation room may not be sterile and I recommend not to use it in the anterior chamber.

Once the A/C is filled with air, complete the surgery and keep the air bubble in the A/C which will be absorbed within 24 hours healing up the Desmet's detachment without any further problem or persistent corneal edema. To reduce this complication, one should limit the number of times that instruments and phaco probe is enters into the anterior chamber.

**Rhexis Run away:**

Misdirection of the anterior capsule during rhexis is a very common problem for the phaco surgeon and more so with the beginners. The corrective steps have been described in the Rhexis section of the book. However, if it is difficult to retrieve a torn rhexis and the margin of the

Capsulorhexis is not continuous, it may be better to convert to SICS to avoid extension of the tear to the equator or to the posterior capsule.

### Constriction of the Pupil and shallow anterior chamber.

After successful start of the surgery, in some cases, the pupil may come down and constrict due to several factors. This is common in Diabetic patients and in others on systemic Flomax and IFIS. If the anterior chamber is shallow at any time, raising the bottle height will deepen the chamber and will allow uneventful surgery.

The corrective measures have been described in the small pupil cases chapter and Floppy Iris syndrome. In diabetic patients, pharmacological agents and Viscoelastics usually allow enough dilatation to complete the surgery. In Floppy Iris Syndrome, one of the mechanical pupil dilating devices may need to be used.

### Rise of Intraocular Pressure During Surgery and positive vitreous pressure:

Increase of Intraocular pressure during surgery in some patients may be caused by positive vitreous pressure to make the anterior chamber shallow, or variation of anterior chamber depth. In obese patients, people with short neck and patients having respiratory disease may show this tendency. Tight Lid Speculum, pull from the drape or low bottle height are other causes of shallow anterior chamber. It is not much difficult to perform Phaco surgery in the presence of moderate amount of increased vitreous pressure. The anterior chamber needs to be filled with viscoelastics every time phaco probe is entered and leave the A/C with irrigation on in foot position 2. Raising the bottle height will increase the depth of the anterior chamber is another important step.

In performing SICS, this is a problem, because increased vitreous pressure bulges the posterior capsule and reduces the space in the anterior chamber and because of a larger incision, it is difficult to keep the anterior chamber formed.

It is better to use Tab. Acetazolamide in the pre operative medication or give an infusion of 200 ml Mannitol iv before surgery in obese patients undergoing SICS. A good akinesia of the eye with local anesthetic reduces intraocular pressure and positive vitreous pressure to facilitate SICS surgery.

If positive vitreous pressure is noted after the surgery is started, the cause may be tight lid speculum or pressure by the drape, try to detect the cause and remove it as soon as possible. Maintain positive pressure in the anterior chamber with viscoelastics and irrigation bottle height raised. After the nucleus is emulsified and epinucleus aspirated, Insertion of the IOL while Posterior capsule is intact and performing I/A for aspiration of the cortex after the IOL is implanted increases safety margin to protect the Posterior capsule from being accidentally injured during these maneuvers.

### Break in the posterior capsule and vitreous loss

**This is the most devastating complication that can occur during cataract surgery.**

Posterior capsular rupture (PCR) and vitreous prolapse occurs in about 1% to 2% of all cataract surgeries. The management requires recognition of the complication early and appropriate measures taken. The risk factors in the preoperative period includes Hypermature cataract, myopia, small pupil, zonular weakness in pseudoexfoliation syndrome, traumatic cataracts, dense asteroid hyalosis and posterior polar cataract. These factors need to be evaluated preoperatively and measures taken to minimize or avoid PCR.

Intraoperatively at each step the risk factors of PCR needs to be recognized as soon this happens so that appropriate corrective measures can be undertaken to minimize the damage.

**During Capsulorhexis:** Radial extension of the rhexis may happen and as soon as the rhexis margin shows tendency to run away, rhexis should be stopped, the anterior chamber is filled with viscoelastic and rhexis started from the opposite direction. If CCC is not achieved, the surgery should be converted to SICS and IOL implanted on the intact posterior capsule. The management of rhexis run away has been discussed in Capsulorhexis section.

**During Hydrodissection:** PCR can happen from over distension of the bag from capsular block due to failure of decompression and fluid trapped under the nucleus. This can be avoided if the surgeon is vigilant. This is more common complication in Posterior Subcapsular and Posterior Polar cataracts.

**During Phacoemulsification:** PCR can happen at any stage of phacoemulsification due to damage to the rhexis margin by the phaco tip or during forceful rotation of the nucleus.

### Signs of Posterior capsule Rupture:

- Sudden dilatation of the pupil
- Sudden deepening of the anterior chamber
- Nuclear fragments do not come towards the phaco tip
- Nucleus do not rotate easily
- Vitreous is visible in anterior chamber.

### Management of the condition depends upon the following factors:

1. Magnitude and size of the posterior capsule tear
2. The amount of nuclear and cortical mater left in the anterior chamber
3. Whether whole or part of the nucleus dropped into the vitreous cavity
4. Whether or not the margin of the Anterior Capsulorhexis is intact

In the case of suspected PCR, it is important not to panic or suddenly come out of the anterior chamber. Sudden movement of anterior chamber may cause extension of the tear and cause more harm than good.

### Steps for management of PCR :

1. Stop the surgery
2. Do not be afraid
3. Do not come out of the anterior chamber abruptly.
4. Do not try to pull at the vitreous
5. Do not introduce instruments into the vitreous to remove fragments
6. Do not do sponge vitrectomy
7. Do not hydrate the vitreous and lower the bottle height but keep the anterior chamber formed at all times.

### Management depends upon the stage of surgery when PCR is detected.

When this happens with nuclear fragments not emulsified, further manipulation of the fragments will cause extension of the PCR. As soon as the PCR is detected, phacoemulsification and aspiration are immediately stopped. Irrigation is continued keeping the foot in Foot Paddle position I. Sudden removal of the foot from the foot paddle will cause the tear to extend further. The phaco probe is kept stable, the second instrument is removed, and viscoelastic is injected through the side port and the anterior chamber is stabilized. **The last instrument to be withdrawn is the phaco probe, without collapsing the anterior chamber. The bottle height is lowered to 20 to 40 cm.**

1. If this is early in the surgical procedure, introduce Viscoelastic to cause temporary tamponade to protect the nucleus from dropping in to the vitreous and convert to SICS. Nucleus is to be removed without pressure on the globe. If the anterior Capsulorhexis is intact and the nucleus is already divided into fragments, enlarge the wound and bring out each fragment using the fish hook, forceps or gentle visco expression.
The cortical clean up is difficult, dry aspiration without irrigation may be performed. The cortical mater may be removed with anterior vitrectomy in closed chamber. Anterior vitrectomy using the vitrectomy probe is performed meticulously to remove all the vitreous strands. A single piece PMMA IOL or Three Piece Foldable IOL may be implanted in the sulcus on the anterior capsule.

2. If PCR is detected while performing hydrodissection, stop the surgery and convert to ECCE and remove the nucleus with vectis after prolapsing it to the anterior chamber. PMMA IOL with big optic 6.5 and overall diameter 13 mm can be implanted in the sulcus on the Anterior capsule after performing anterior vitrectomy.

3. If the PCR is small and occurs late in the surgery when cortical aspiration has been done or almost done, the main wound should be closed by a suture and anterior vitrectomy is performed using vitreous cutter. The IOL to be implanted depends upon the size of the Posterior capsule Tear and the size of the anterior Capsulorhexis. A Foldable IOL can be implanted on the anterior capsule if the original rhexis was 5 mm and a 7 mm Optic Foldable IOL is available. Otherwise, a single piece PMMA Lens is preferred to be placed in the sulcus.

**Complications related to Posterior Capsule Rupture:**

1. Vitreous traction and retinal break
2. Retinal Detachment
3. Macular Edema (CME)
4. Uveitis and Vitritis
5. IOL displacement
6. Endophthalmitis.

The occurrence of PCR is a dreaded complication and can occur at any stage of cataract surgery. It is important for the cataract surgeon to recognize the PCR early and corrective measures taken to avoid serious complications like retinal detachment. All the post operative complications result from inadequate removal of vitreous and traction at the vitreous base. As soon as the PCR is detected, phacoemulsification and aspiration are immediately stopped. The anterior chamber is stabilized as described and preparation is taken to convert the surgery as appropriate. It is important to detect early and corrective measures taken to avoid further complications.

**Anterior Vitrectomy using bimanual procedure:**

Vitrectomy requires a vitreous cutter handpiece and an irrigation line. All phaco machines are equipped with an anterior vitrectomy handpiece and a vitrectomy port. The vitrectomy probe is attached to the phaco machine and the mode is selected. The phaco incision is closed with one suture. A new side port incision is created.

The infusion line is placed through the original side port with a low bottle height. The cutter is passed through the second side port thus the surgery is performed through a closed system. A high cut rate and low flow are chosen. The cutting rate should be set at the highest rate on the phaco machine, and vacuum of 100 mm Hg to 150 mm Hg is adequate. Traction on retina during cutting and removal of vitreous is minimum at this setting.

Triamcinolone acetonide (Kenalog Bristol Myers Squibb) 40 mg/ ml is injected into the anterior chamber. The white product sticks to the vitreous and makes it visible and it is easy to remove this by the vitrectomy cutter.

The vitrectomy cutter probe is placed through the PCR with the cutting port positioned behind the posterior capsule. Anterior vitreous is thus removed. The cutter is then moved forward into the capsular bag to remove the remaining lens matter with the cut rate at 300 cpm. The cortex is removed next, using the vacuum-only setting of the cutter, while the cutting action is stopped. The cortex is freed and drawn into the center, and the cutting action is activated to remove it. Thus the anterior chamber is made free of any vitreous and cortical mater. The anterior chamber is filled with viscoelastic and the irrigation port is withdrawn.

The main phaco incision is now opened by removing the suture. If there is adequate anterior capsular support, implantation of an IOL into the ciliary sulcus is possible. The overall diameter of the chosen IOL should be at least 13 mm. and optic size bigger than the anterior Capsulorhexis. Single Piece PMMA IOL or Multi piece Foldable IOL may be used for implantation in the sulcus. In case of small central tear that can be converted into a posterior capsulorhexis, in-the-bag implantation is also possible.

The viscoelastic is next removed and pupil is constricted using Miochol or non preserved Pilocarpine. Wound integrity is checked and if any leak is noted, the wound is closed with one or two 10/0 Nylon suture with the ends buried into the corneal stroma.

The cataract surgeon must learn anterior vitrectomy technique before attempting phaco surgery. Practicing on cadaver eyes or goats eyes to perform vitrectomy correctly is important and to be mastered. Although we do not expect this serious and dreadful complication to happen, but cataract surgeons have to face this situation at some point and effective management with good surgical technique and postoperative care will in most cases bring good visual outcome.

Never attempt to do sponge vitrectomy because, the vitreous is like a slinky and if pulled, more and more vitreous comes out and will stick to the wound, iris and other structures. Never chase the nuclear fragments with vectis or other instruments. This will cause more disruption of the vitreous and more vitreous loss.

## NUCLEUS DROP: POSTERIOR DISLOCATION OF NUCLEUS:

Nucleus drop or posterior dislocation of nucleus or nucleus fragments is another difficult complication. If the nucleus fragments are seen to get displaced posteriorly, injection of Viscoelastic behind the nucleus fragment may stop further dropping and the fragment may be removed using the techniques described. However, if the nucleus or nuclear fragment continues to drop posteriorly, this should never be chased by vectis, phaco probe or any other instrument. It is dangerous even trying to remove nuclear fragments from the vitreous cavity using vectis and may cause retinal detachment. Treat it as a posterior capsule rupture and vitreous loss case. It is safer to manage the anterior segment as described above and implant the IOL. Leave any posteriorly dislocated nuclear fragments or the whole nucleus for a vitreo-retina specialist to deal with. This will require a separate surgery by pars plana posterior vitrectomy and removal of the nucleus fragment. Leaving the nuclear fragment for a long period of time in the vitreous will cause inflammation and cystoid macular edema (CME) and must be removed as soon as possible by the vitreo-retina specialist.

**References :**

1. Lundström M, Behndig A, Montan P, et al. Capsule complication during cataract surgery: Background, study design, and required additional care: Swedish Capsule Rupture Study Group report 1. J Cataract Refract Surg. 2009;37(10):1762-1767.

2. Packard R. Technique prevents nucleus drop through capsular tear. Ocular Surgery News. 2001;19:14

3. Burk SE, Da Mata AP, Snyder ME, Schneider S, Osher RH, Cionni RJ. Visualizing vitreous using kenalog suspension. J Cataract Refract Surg. 2003;29(4):645-651.

4. Spigelman AV, Lindstrom RL, Nichols BD, Lindquist TD. Visual results following vitreous loss and primary lens implantation. J Cataract Refract Surg. 1989;15(2):201-204.

5. Tano Y, Chandler D, Machemer R. Treatment of intraocular proliferation with intravitreal injection of triamcinolone acetonide. Am J Ophthalmol. 1980;90(6):810-816.

6. McCuen BW 2nd, Bessler M, Tano Y, Chandler D, Machemer R. The lack of toxicity of intravitreally administered triamcinolone acetonide. Am J Ophthalmol. 1981;91(6):785-788.

7. Hida T, Chandler D, Arena JE, Machemer R. Experimental and clinical observations of the intraocular toxicity of commercial corticosteroid preparations. Am J Ophthalmol. 1986 Feb 15;101(2):190-5.

8. Young S, Larkin G, Branley M, Lightman S. Safety and efficacy of intravitreal triamcinolone for cystoid macular oedema in uveitis. Clin Experiment Ophthalmol. 2001;29(1):2-6.

9. Peyman GA, Cheema R, Conway MD, Fang T. Triamcinolone acetonide as an aid to visualization of the vitreous and the posterior hyaloid during pars plana vitrectomy. Retina. 2000;20(5):554-555.

10. Osher R, Cionni R. The torn posterior capsule: Its intra-operative behavior, surgical management, and long-term consequences. J Cataract Refract Surg. 1990;16:490-494.

11. Horiguchi M, Miyake K, Ohta I, Ito Y. Staining of the lens capsule for circular continuous capsulorhexis in eyes with white cataract. Arch Ophthalmol. 1998;116(4):535-537

# Chapter 17
# POST OPERATIVE COMPLICATIONS

Post operative complications after cataract surgery is an undesirable event and can largely be prevented. Recognition of the complication at the earliest opportunity and appropriate and decisive treatment will cure most of the complications. We will describe post operative complications by structures affected starting anteriorly to the retina posteriorly.

1. **Conjunctiva** :

   1.1 **Conjunctivitis** due to bacteria or virus may happen during the immediate postoperative period. It is desirable to prevent this by isolating the patient should such an infective focus is detected in the household. However, after phacoemulsification the corneal wound is self sealing and should conjunctivitis be detected at any time during the postoperative period, this should be treated energetically with standard medications which usually heals up completely. Topical corticosteroids should be stopped or reduced since spread of infection may lead to endophthalmitis.

   1.2 **Giant Papillary Conjunctivitis:** This is usually due to trauma to the palpebral conjunctiva by suture ends. Exposed suture ends that are not buried in the cornea or under conjunctiva may cause granulomatous inflammation of the palpebral conjunctiva. The patient complains of intermittent blurring of vision, foreign body sensation, ropy discharge and hemorrhage.

   Management of the condition is to remove or trim the suture ends, Topical antibiotics, steroids and lubricating drops as frequently as required. Complete resolution takes about three to four weeks.

2. **Corneal Complications** :

   2.1 **Dry cornea due to exposure:** The cornea may be cloudy due to exposure during surgery if enough BSS drops or viscoelastic are not applied on the surface of the cornea. If this happens, the epithelium becomes hazy and subsequent surgical steps may become difficult. On completion of the surgery, an antibiotic ointment is applied and bandage or bandage contact lens applied. The cornea becomes clear once the epithelium is healed.

   2.2 **Punctuate Epithelial Lesions (SPK):** SPK following surgery is usually due to toxic effect of topical eye drops. The superficial corneal epithelial lesions appear one to two weeks after cataract surgery. Some medications like Benzalkonium Chloride, Beta Blockers, steroids and in fact any eye drops can cause SPK. Patients presents with decreased vision, a red eye and foreign body sensation.

Slit lamp examination reveals diffuse injection of the conjunctiva and punctate staining in the central corneal epithelium with fluorescein dye. If the staining is uniform, punctate staining can usually be appreciated when excess fluorescein dye is irrigated out from the eye.

Management consists of withdrawal of the offending eye drop and frequent use of topical non preserved artificial tears and lubricating eye drops. Any other eye drops to be used during the entire postoperative period must be preservative free.

Special care is required in the treatment of patients with severe ocular surface disease, because the use of medications toxic to the epithelium, especially nonsteroidal anti-inflammatory drugs (NSAIDs), in conjunction with topical steroids can lead to corneal ulceration.

The cases should be frequently followed up until complete resolution which takes about 3 to 4 weeks.

**2.3 Corneal Injury:** Corneal injury due to accidental or self induced trauma may happen during postoperative period and should be managed by standard procedures.

**2.4 Corneal Stromal Edema:** Stromal edema is mainly due to endothelial injury during surgery. Phacoemulsification generates heat and turbulence in the anterior chamber that can cause damage to endothelial cells leading to stromal edema ranging from striate keratopathy to deep corneal clouding and decompensation.

**Causes of persistent corneal edema: a)** Endothelial damage during surgery, b) Retained Cortical or Nuclear fragments in the anterior chamber, c) Prolonged inflammation d) Persistent rise of Intraocular Pressure.

Management consists of grading the edema, lubricating eye drops and steroids in cases of mild striate keratopathy. Striate keratopathy resolves in about two to three weeks. Deep corneal edema requires a Bandage contact lens, Hypertonic Saline eye drops and topical steroid eye drops. It may take long time and may be difficult to resolve. Unresolved corneal edema causing decompensation requires a Corneal Transplant

**2.5 Corneal Endothelial injury:**

Corneal endothelium is assaulted during phaco surgery in many ways and these results in loss of some endothelial cells during the surgery. Significant number of endothelial cell loss depends on some factors:

a)      Preoperative status of the corneal endothelial cell count

b)      Surgical trauma

c)      Type of IOL implantation

d)      Post operative complications

**2.5.1.** Preoperative status of corneal endothelium must be assessed and documented. Pre existing disease like Fuch's Dystrophy, Diabetes and Corneal Guttata needs to be evaluated properly and in all cases of doubt, a Specular Microscopy and record of endothelial cell count obtained before surgery. If Specular Microscopy is not available, the surgeon must examine the corneal endothelium under magnification and explain the possibility of outcome to the patient. This also requires the surgeon to be careful during surgery to minimize trauma to the endothelium and protect the same with good Viscoelastic.

The cornea may develop pseudophakic bullous keratopathy after cataract surgery, once the endothelial cell function and the endothelial cell population have been reduced to a significant low level. A cell count of less than 400 per square millimeters, pachymetry reading of more than 650 μm, morning edema, or loose epithelium may signal imminent decompensation of the cornea.

**2.5.2. Surgical Trauma:** It has been documented that continuous irrigation of anterior chamber with BSS for 30 minutes does not cause significant endothelial cell loss in experimental animals. However, during Phaco surgery some endothelial cells are lost due to the heat and turbulence created in the anterior chamber by the vibrating Phaco tip. Utmost care is to be taken to protect the endothelium with good quality viscoelastics throughout surgery and during all instrumentation in the anterior chamber. The space in the anterior chamber is a few mm and all the movements of the phaco tip to break and emulsify the nucleus has to be performed within this confined space. Performing phaco in the anterior chamber for any reason is dangerous and causes endothelial cell loss and some corneal edema. Phaco energy must be delivered away from the corneal endothelium and all instruments and IOL must be handled in such a way that they do not touch the corneal endothelium. Turbulence of nuclear fragments inside the A/C is also dangerous and causes damage to the cornea. Loss of endothelial cells may be caused by sudden collapse of the anterior chamber and touch with the phaco tip or IOL during insertion.

**2.5.3 Type of Intraocular Lens:** Corneal endothelial cell loss is also documented after certain type of IOL implantation. Iris supported IOL (not used now) and AC IOL (rarely used) is associated with cell loss in the short and long term. PC IOL if not implanted in the bag, may cause endothelial cell loss. Foldable IOL implanted in the bag is not likely to cause significant endothelial cell loss unless the lens rubs on the endothelium during implantation.

**2.5.4 :Post Operative Complications :** Rise of intraocular pressure, presence of inflammation, retained cortical mater and anterior capsular fragments on the endothelium may give rise to corneal edema and endothelial cell loss. All these complications can be prevented by meticulous cleaning the anterior chamber at the end of the surgery.

**2.5.5. Retrocorneal Membranes**

Appearance of a retrocorneal membranes in the postoperative period is a rare event. These membranes may appear as fine gray lines on the posterior corneal surface and have pigmentation associated with them. The cause of formation of a retrocorneal membrane may be :

a) Epithelial ingrowth (epithelial cysts)

b) Stromal Ingrowth

c) Corneal endothelial overgrowth

d) Peripheral anterior synechia

e) Iris melanocytosis

Management of the condition depends upon the cause and either conservative management or surgical excision is advised. This is rare now due to clear corneal incisions in phaco surgery.

**2.6 Corneal Melting**

A patient who initially presents with punctate corneal staining, which becomes an epithelial defect, may ultimately develop stromal loss. The majority of these patients do not complain of pain. Rheumatoid arthritis; scleroderma, Stevens-Johnson's syndrome, radiation and collagen vascular disease may be associated with corneal melting.

The differential diagnosis for corneal ulceration following IOL implantation includes all the usual causes of this problem. Microbial keratitis - including bacterial, fungal, amoebic, and viral etiologies - should be ruled out by appropriate laboratory studies.

Rheumatoid arthritis, Wegener granulomatosis, Sjögren syndrome, malnutrition, hypovitaminosis-A, Mooren ulcer, or a marginal ulcer secondary to blepharitis should be considered.

Management of the condition is difficult and consists of, frequent lubrication with a nonpreserved drop or ointment should be instituted and the patient should be hospitalized. Bandage contact lenses, Corneal cyanoacrylate glue and Tarsorraphy has been advocated. Healing results in approximately 60% of these cases. Spontaneous perforation should be treated with either a lamellar or penetrating keratoplasty or conjunctival hood. **Autologous serum 10 times a day and Amniotic membrane graft may be considered.**

### 2.7. CORNEAL ULCER:

Corneal Ulcer may complicate cataract surgery. Acute traumatic, bacterial, viral, or fungal ulcers will usually produce pain and a prominent inflammatory reaction and emergency treatment is required to prevent corneal opacity and other sight threatening complications to develop.

a) Traumatic ulcers are usually sterile unless contaminated and should be treated by conservative measures with antibiotics, bandage contact lens and cycloplegics. All steroid and NSID drops should be stopped.

b) Fungal corneal ulcers are dangerous, and should be suspected if there is a history of vegetative trauma. Treatment consists of antifungal agents, cycloplegics and examination of corneal scraping by gram stain and giemsa stain.

c) Bacterial corneal ulcer should be appropriately treated with corneal scraping culture sensitivity and institution of broad spectrum antibiotics and cycloplegics, a subconjunctival injection of antibiotics should be considered.

d) HSV and other viral corneal ulcer may complicate cataract surgery especially in elderly and immunocompromised or diabetic patients. Immediate stopping of steroids and treatment with acyclovir ointment five times a day, cycloplegics and lubricating drops usually brings complete resolution.

In all cases of corneal ulcer, the patient is to be monitored very closely for intraocular inflammation and healing of the ulcer.

### 3. Flat Anterior Chamber

Flat or shallow anterior chamber in the immediate postoperative period may be due to Wound Leak or Choroidal Detachment.

Wound leak occurs due to inadequate closure of the wound and is diagnosed by a positive Seidel Test which is performed by installation of one drop Fluorescein in the conjunctival sac and dilution of the dye at the site of leak is visible on Slit Lamp. The Intraocular Pressure is low and may cause choroidal effusion.

Closure of the wound with sutures, cycloplegics, and application of pad and Bandage reforms the anterior chamber within 24 hours. On rare occasions, the A/C may need to be reformed surgically by BSS or air introduced in the anterior chamber.

4. **Micro Hyphaema Syndrome :** Small hemorrhage may occur in the immediate postoperative period or may present 6 weeks to 2 years after surgery. On examination, blood cells or ghost cells may be present in the anterior chamber. The condition is very often overlooked because, by the time the patient comes to the doctor's office, the hyphaema is absorbed. This complication may rarely be seen in Sulcus Fixated IOL causing erosion of the angle by the lens loop and any complain of blurring of vision or pain in the post operative period should be examined critically. Management of the condition is with cycloplegics, topical steroid-antibiotic eye drops. This is cured within one week but may recur.

5. **High Intraocular Pressure:**

   5.1 **Known Glaucoma:** Preexisting glaucoma must be treated before surgery with medications to control IOP. Phaco surgery reduces IOP and management of glaucoma is described in the chapter cataract with Glaucoma.

   5.2 **Rise of Intraocular Pressure in the immediate postoperative period:**

   The Intraocular pressure may increase following surgery sometimes in the region of 40 to 60 mm Hg. This transient rise of IOP is due to retained viscoelastics or cortical mater. The rise of intraocular pressure in the immediate postoperative period may cause damage to the optic nerve and is more severe if there is preexisting glaucoma. The viscoelastics and cortical mater must be cleared as far as possible at the end of surgery. If there is doubt, one tab Acetazolamide in the evening and one tab in the morning the following day should be given. Intraocular pressure must be measured at each post operative visit and if high IOP is detected at any time during the first post operative week, IOP lowering treatment must be started immediately. This consists of oral agents like Acetazolamide, topical beta blockers and if the IOP is very high, Mannitol infusion. The induced intraocular pressure is usually controlled within one week and the medications should be withdrawn gradually.

**5.3 Pupillary Block Glaucoma:** Pupillary block is rare event. This may happen if there are inflammatory exudates to block the pupil. Dilatation of the pupil with mydriatic/cycloplegic drops, control of inflammation with topical and systemic steroids will control the rise of IOP. If necessary, one may consider YAG LASER Peripheral Iridectomy and Mannitol infusion to reduce the intraocular pressure quickly.

**5.4 Steroid Induced Glaucoma:** Prolonged use of steroids in the post operative period especially in young and susceptible patients may give rise to steroid induced glaucoma. The condition should be detected and treated immediately to avoid any damage to the optic nerve. Treatment consists of, stopping topical steroid drops immediately and substitution with Non- steroidal anti-inflammatory agents and weak steroid drops like fluorometholone and concomitant use of anti glaucoma medications. The IOP must be monitored closely and adequately controlled.

**5.5 Secondary Glaucoma:** Secondary Glaucoma due to blockage of the angle with inflammatory exudates or formation Peripheral anterior Synechiae is rare event but is possible. This should be kept in mind and managed if detected in the post operative period.

6. **Precipitates on the IOL: Precipitates** may be observed on the IOL in cases which runs a course of prolonged inflammation. The cells may be pigmented and may be deposition of, macrophages, giant cells and histocytes. These deposits do not cause any harm unless associated with iritis or CME. If either of these conditions is present, appropriate anti inflammatory treatment is to be started; otherwise these may be left alone. I have found some cases where application of low intensity YAG LASER may disperse these cells and later absorbed.

7. **MALPOSITION OF POSTERIOR CHAMBER LENS.**

After placement of the posterior chamber lens in position, the lens may be decentrated, dislocated or even lost. It is important to understand the reasons & corrective measures taken to avoid them.

**7.1. Optic Decentration:**

Some amount of optic decent ration may be present in sulcus fixated IOL.

It is best to dial the lens to bring the loops in the horizontal position. Significant decentration is termed when the edge of the optic is in the pupillary space. Patients complain of glare and occasional blurring of vision.

**7.2. Malpositioned Loop** : The loops may be malpositioned, one in the bag, the other in the sulcus and this causes slight tilting of the lens & no symptoms. More serious malposition causes lens lilt. This may cause iris atrophy & recurrent mild inflammation & microhyphaema.

### 7.3. WINDSHIELD WIPER SYNDROME:

This is a situation where the inferior loop is fixed and stable in the bag. But the upper loop & optic rocks from side to side superiorly in the sulcus.

This occurs due to a short overall diameter lens that is in a comparatively longer eyeball. The patient complains of glare and reduced vision and occasional blurring.

Management of the condition consists of exchange the lens and rotation of the lens in horizontal position. When the lens is placed in the bag this complication is avoided.

### 7.4. SUNRISE SYNDROME:

In this situation, the IOL is displaced superiorly.

The most common cause is placement of a PC IOL with one loop in the bag and the other loop in the sulcus. Usually, the inferior loop is in the bag and the superior loop in the sulcus or, both the loops are in the sulcus. If there is zonular dehiscence, the superior loop protrudes through the dehiscence & this causes dragging the superior loop upwards.

Usually the patient has no complaints unless the displacement is so severe that the lens displaces out of the visual axis. If the displacement is symptomless, nothing needs to be done. If the displacement is severe, reposition of the lens is indicated. If there is big zonular disinsertion, the management becomes more difficult. Lens exchange can be performed.

### 7.5. SUNSET SYNDROME

This is a somewhat difficult situation. The lens dislocates interiorly through a zonular dehiscence downwards. It may continue to descend or may stop descending because of fibrosis and fixation of the other loop. However, this is a recognized complication and can be prevented in two ways. Firstly in the bag placement of IOL reduces the risk of zonular disinsertion and the other is rotation & dialing the lens in horizontal position in the sulcus. Should this complication occur, my recommended management would be reposition of the lens or removal of the IOL & replacement by a bigger optic size lens.

**7.6. LOST LENS SYNDROME :**

This is an extension of the sunset syndrome or may occur due to trauma. The lens may dislocate & be lost in the vitreous cavity or may be extruded from the eye through a traumatic rupture of the wound.

I encountered few such cases only. One patient sustained a blunt trauma to the eye 6 weeks post-operatively and the lens dislocated into the vitreous. On another occasion, during dental extraction, due to the jerk or force applied, the posterior capsule was torn and the lens dropped into the vitreous in previously asymptomatic patient.

My recommended management of a lost lens syndrome is to refer the patient to a vitreo-retina surgeon who will remove the IOL after vitrectomy & implant a sulcus fixated IOL. Unfortunately, in both the cases, although the lens was removed by the vitreo retina surgeon, the patients did not get back useful vision.

## 8. POST OPERATIVE IRIS COMPLICATIONS:

**8.1. PROTRACTED UVEITIS :** Some inflammation in the postoperative period is expected. However, severe post operative inflammation is to be treated as endophthalmitis.

**8.2. OVALLING OF THE IRIS:** Rarely seen today this used to be a major complication with A/C IOL

Implantation. Because of iris –lens touch and fibroblastic activity, the Pupil would be pulled and assume an oval shape. This complication is not seen with Posterior Camber IOL implant.

**8.3 IRIS CHAFING :** Iris may be injured during phacoemulsification and patchy areas of iris tissue loss is seen. This may cause transillumination defect. This does not interfere with vision. If inflammation is present, this may be treated with topical steroids and NSID drops.

## 9. CYSTOID MACULAR EDEMA: 
Post operative cystoid macular edema occurs in all types of eye surgeries and is common cause of reduced visual acuity in the post operative period. Post operative CME is also known as Irvine-Gass Syndrome. The condition is further described at a separate chapter.

## 10. ENDOPHTHALMITIS : 
Severe Inflammation in the post operative period is called Endophthalmitis.

This is the most devastating post operative complication and is sight threatening. Management of endophthalmitis is a challenge and special measures are to be undertaken to prevent and manage this dreadful condition. This is described in a separate chapter.

**11. RETINAL DETACHMENT :** Pseudophakic retinal detachment occurs infrequently and is common in patients having preoperative risk factors. These patients need to be identified and closely monitored.

**Predisposing factors for retinal detachment are:**

a)   **Retinal Detachment in the fellow eye**
b)   **High Myopia**
c)   **Posterior capsule opening as a surgical complication of PCR or YAG LASER PCT**
d)   **Vitreous loss due to posterior capsule rupture or ICCE**
e)   **Diabetes Mellitus**
f)   **Peripheral Retinal Degenerations**

Retinal detachment is a possibility wherever there is a history of recent significant reduction of visual acuity and a history of flashes and floaters. Any patient complaining of floater and flashes of light must be examined with an indirect ophthalmoscope and any weak points in the retina with traction identified and treated. A complaint of Flashes of light and Floaters should never be ignored.

Should retinal detachment happen in a Pseudophakic eye, the management is the same as in any other retinal detachment patient. Prompt hospitalization, referral to a vitreo-retina surgeon & early surgery saves vision.

High risk patients like High Myopes, Retinal detachment in the fellow eye and patients having vitreous loss should be closely followed up. Patients should be warned about the pre-monitoring symptoms of retinal detachment. Patients with diabetes mellitus may get a traction retinal detachment as a part of proliferative Diabetic retinopathy and should be managed accordingly.

## 12. POSTERIOR CAPSULAR OPACITY

Opacification of the posterior capsule remains the most frequent complication of cataract surgery.

Most cases of clinical PCO are caused by the proliferation of residual epithelial cells left in the capsular bag following cataract surgery and classic PCO are caused by proliferation of the equatorial cells.

Actually, it is not the capsule that opacifies, rather, an opaque membrane develops as retained cells proliferate and migrate onto the posterior capsular surface.

The interval between surgery and PCO varies, ranging anywhere from 3 months to 4 years after the surgery. The causes of PCO are multifactorial as reported in several studies, younger patients gets PCO earlier than the older age group. Several factors have been held responsible for PCO formation. The factors are, Neurofibroblastic differentiation of epithelial cells, remnants of residual epithelial cells causing migration of cells over the posterior capsule, growth of cells from the anterior capsule and posterior capsule touch and remnants of cortical mater that form pearls or fibrous bands on the posterior capsule. In the normal anatomic situation, the lens epithelial cells are found at the anterior surface at the equatorial region and the equatorial lens bow. This is a single row of cuboidal cells that can proliferate and produce PCO.

a)  The anterior- zone under the anterior lens capsule consists of a single layer of flat cuboidal, epithelial cells with minimal mitotic activity. These anterior epithelial cells ("A" cells) proliferate and undergo fibrous metaplasia to produce the posterior capsular opacity and anterior capsular contraction.

b)  The formation of Soemmering's ring and Elsings Pearls around the lens equator is due to proliferation of the E cells. This layer is a continuation of anterior lens cells around the equator, forming the equatorial lens bow ("E" cells). While the A cells are inactive, the E cells show cell mitoses, division, and multiplication and are active thus, new lens fibers are continuously produced in this zone throughout life. Proliferation of these cells causes more dense opacities and pearls.

Whatever be the mechanism of formation of PCO, this reduces vision and once formed needs removal to restore vision. Irrespective of the factors causing Posterior Capsule Opacity, the patients complain of glare, reduced visual acuity and reduced ability to see near objects.

**Management of Posterior Capsule Opacity:**

a)  **Surgical Posterior Capsulotomy:** Where YAG LASER facility is not available, Posterior capsulotomy can be performed surgically using a knife or needle. Under local anesthesia, a needle is passed under the lens aiming the center of the capsule under direct visualization.

A triangular cut in the posterior capsule is made and postoperatively steroids and actazolamide is prescribed.

**b)** **YAG LASER POSTERIOR CAPSULOTOMY :**

**Nd YAG LASER is most frequently used to perform posterior capsulotomy.** A Q SWITHCHED

ND YAG LASER with Slit Lamp attachment is adequate.

The procedure is performed under topical anesthesia. A small capsulotomy centered at the pupil and the size slightly bigger than the pupil should be performed. The center of the pupil is marked, the pupil is dilated. Use of a contact lens is optional. The Laser is focused accurately on the Posterior capsule and capsulotomy is performed with minimum power which is adequate to cut the capsule. Disruption of vitreous using high energy is undesirable and is to be avoided. Post operatively, topical Steroids and one tab Acetazolamide is usually adequate, optional use of beta blocker is indicated if the IOP is expected to be high.

This is an out - patient procedure but may be associated with the following complications:

1. Elevation of Intraocular Pressure
2. IOL optic damage : IOL Pitting
3. Retinal detachment
4. Cystoid Macular Edema
5. IOL Crack
6. IOL subluxation
7. Corneal Endothelial damage
8. Vitreous prolapse in the anterior chamber

Timing of the YAG LASER procedure is Important. In general, it is better not to perform YAG Laser capsulotomy earlier than three months after surgery and can be performed at any time thereafter.

Several procedures have been described and research has been performed to prevent Posterior Capsular opacification (PCO) but an uniform procedure has not yet been recommended.

## 13. PAIN AND GLARE :

Some patients may complain of pain any time after surgery. Never dismiss a complaint of pain.

Pain in the immediate post-operative patient may be due to uveitis, rise of intraocular pressure and

Endophthalmitis. It is important to examine the patient with a Slit lamp & appropriate therapy should be started immediately. Episcleritis & Scleritis may be the cause of pain and should be treated with appropriate medications including NSID and steroids.

Sometimes the patient may complain of unexplainable pain 3 to 6 months after surgery. On examination nothing may be found wrong but a very mild flare and cells in the anterior chamber may be observed. This happens due to erosion of the ciliary body by the lens loops when the IOL is implanted in the sulcus. Management of this condition is intermittent use of steroid drops if the visual acuity is stable. The pain may disappear over a period of time when the lens is fixed in the sulcus by fibrosis.

If there is decrease of visual acuity and pain, this may be due to several other factors including CME or iris neovascularization. In these situations, appropriate management of the cause is indicated.

**My advice is, don't ignore the complaint of pain and specially a deep aching pain in the eye-ball in Pseudophakic patients. Keep a close watch and manage them appropriately.**

Some patients may complain of Migraine like symptoms long after a lens implant. They should be evaluated by a neurologist. Standard treatment for migraine can then be initiated.

Glaucoma & low grade iritis must be excluded-in all these patients. It is not uncommon to find patients who complain of glare. This results from scattering of light entering the eye. Various factors are responsible for glare in a patient with an IOL implant. They include optic decentration, posterior capsule Opacification, pupil size and many other factors. These patients should be examined thoroughly and if

causative factor can be identified; appropriate treatment is to be given. If no cause is found and the patient has good visual acuity, reassurance is enough. However, if this becomes distressing to the patients, repositioning or exchange IOL may be considered.

## 14. NEGATIVE DYSPHOTOPSIA

Negative Dysphotopsia is a rare complain of the patients after IOL implantation who see flickering of light in their temporal field of vision. This is associated with acrylic lens implantation and almost always resolves over a period of time. If troublesome, miotic eye drops may be prescribed and patient reassured. If all management fails, a lens exchange with a bigger optic size may be required.

**REFERENCES :**

1. Insler MS, Boutros GM, Boulware DW. Corneal ulceration following cataract surgery in patients with rheumatoid arthritis. *Am Intraocular Implant Soc J.* 1985;11:594-597.

2. Yang HK, Kline OR. Corneal melting with intraocular lenses. *Arch Ophthalmol.* 1982;100:1272-1274.

3. Gelender H. Descemetocele after intraocular lens implantation. *Arch Ophthalmol.* 1982;100:72-76.

4. Moses L. Localized bullous keratopathy secondary to adherent lens capsule. *Arch Ophthalmol.* 1986;104:639-640.

5. Vastine DW, Weinberg RS, Surger J, Binder PS. Stripping of Descemet's membrane associated with intraocular lens implantation. *Arch Ophthalmol.* 1983;101:1042-1045.

6. Bourne WM, Kaufman HE. Endothelial damage associated with intraocular lenses. *Am J Ophthalmol.* 1976;81:482-485

7. Kaufman HE, Katz JI. Endothelial damage from intraocular lens insertion. *Invest Ophthalmol.* 1976;15:996.

8. Forstot SL, Blackwell WL, Jaffe NS, Kaufman HE. The effect of intraocular lens implantation on the corneal endothelium. *Ophthalmol/Otolarynogol.* 1977;83:195-203.

9. Sugar J, Mitchelson J, Kraff M. Endothelial trauma and cell intraocular lens insertion. *Arch Ophthalmol.* 1978;96:449-450.

10. Aron-Rosa D, Cohn HC, Aron JJ, Boquety C. Methylcellulose instead of Healon in extracapsular surgery with intraocular lens implantation. *Am Acad Ophthalmol.* 1983;90:1235-1238.

11. McCarey BE, Polack FM, Marshall W. The phacoemulsification procedure. Part I: The effect of intraocular irrigating solutions on the corneal endothelium. *Invest Ophthalmol.* 1976;15:449-457.

12. Binder PS, Sternberg H, Wickham MG, Worthen DM. Corneal endothelial damage associated with phacoemulsification. *Am J Ophthalmol.* 1976;82(1):48-54.

13. Waltman SRS, Cozean CH. The effect of phacoemulsification on the endothelium. *Ophthalmic Surg.* 1979;10:31-33.

14. Beesley RD, Olson JJ, Brady SE. The effects of prolonged phacoemulsification time on the corneal endothelium. *An Ophthalmol.* 1986;18:216-222.

15. Kraff MC, Sanders DR, Lieberman HL. Specular microscopy in cataract and intraocular lens patients: A report of 564 cases. *Arch Ophthalmol.* 1980;98:1782-1784.

16. Essentials of Cataract and Lens Implant Surgery, Dr. SMMunirul Huq, Karl Holzinger Jesmine publications, Dhaka, 1977.

17. Kaufman HE: Cataract extraction on mild and severe guttata cases. Welsh R.C., Welsh J (Ed.): *The New Report on Cataract Surgery, Proceedings of the First Cataract Surgical Congress*, Miami, Fla., Miami Educational Press, Inc., 1969:187-

18. Drews RC. Intermittent touch syndrome. *Arch Ophthalmol.* 1982;100:1440-1412

19. Liesegang TJ, Bourne WM, Ilstrup DM. Short-and long-term endothelial cell loss associated with cataract extraction and intraocular lens implantation. *Am J Ophthalmol.* 1984;97:32-39.

20. Feder RS, Krachmer JH. Diagnosis of epithelial downgrowth after keratoplasty. *Am J Ophthalmol.* 1985;99:697-703.

21. Richburg FA. Neodymium:YAG laser for anterior capsulotomy. *Am Intraocular Implant Soc J.* 1985;11(4):372-375.

22. Rowsey JJ, Gaylor JR. Intraocular lens disasters: Peripheral anterior synechia. *Ophthalmology.* 1980;87:646-664.

23. Holweger RR, Marefat B. Intraocular pressure change after Neodymium:YAG capsulotomy. J Cataract Refract Surg. 1997;23(1):115-21.

24. Masket S (Eds). Cataract Surgery In Complicated Cases, orofare NJ: Slack Inc; lOOO. pp 399-417

25. Pandey SK, Ram J, Werner L, et al. Visual results and postoperative complications of capsular bag versus sulcus fixation of posterior chamber intraocular lenses for traumatic cataract in children. J Cataract Refract Surg. 1999;25(12): 1576-84.

26. Apple DJ, Peng Q, Visessook N, et al. Eradication of posterior capsular opacification. Documentation of a marked decrease in Nd:YAG laser posterior capsulotomy rates noted in an analysis of 5416 pseudophakic human eyes obtained postmortem. Ophthalmology. 2001;108(3):505-18.

27. Font RL, Brownstein S. A light and electron microscopic study of anterior subcapsular cataracts. Am J Ophthalmol. 1974;78(6):972-84.

28. Apple DJ, Peng Q, Visessook N, et al. Surgical prevention of posterior capsular opacification. Part I. Progress in eliminating this complication of cataract surgery. J Cataract Refract Surg. 2000;26(2): 180- 7.

29. Richter CU, Steinert RF. Neodymium: Yttrium Aluminium Garnet laser posterior capsulotomy. In: SteinertRF (Ed). Cataract Surgery: Techniques, Complications and Management. Philadelphia, PA: WB Saunders Company; 1995. pp 378-8.

30. Koch D, Liu J, Gill P, et al. Axial myopia increases the risk of retinal complications after Neodymium-YAG laser posterior capsulotomy. Arch Ophthalmol. 1989;107(7):986-90.

31. Apple DJ, Solomon KD, Tetz MR, et al. Posterior capsular opacification. Surv Ophthalmol. 1992;37(2):73-116.

# Chapter 18

# POST OPERATIVE ENDOPHTHALMITIS

Post operative endophthalmitis is a devastating and most distressing complication of cataract surgery and can be associated with any form of intraocular surgery. The incidence of this complication has reduced with modern techniques. Present quoted incidence rate ranges from 0.13% to 0.7% after cataract surgery, of which culture positive infectious endophthalmitis accounts for approximately 70% of cases and Sterile Endophthalmitis in 30%cases. Endogenous Endophthalmitis can also occur in diabetic and immunocompromised patients. Endophthalmitis is a sight threatening condition and therefore the surgeon must be able to recognize it at the earliest stage and manage the case with competence so that the damage done is minimized. However, it is an undesirable condition in the postoperative period and the first reaction of the surgeon is that of horror, and the terrified surgeon must retain all the wits to treat the complication rather than avoid it. **Every ophthalmic surgeon should be prepared to come across and manage Endophthalmitis sometime in clinical life, and when confronted, must act promptly to save the eye.** When this complication occurs, the surgeon must have a clear and logical set of protocol for the management of the condition in mind. It is more important for the surgeon to prevent endophthalmitis by maintaining high standards and protocols for the operating theatre and the ancillary facilities.

**Classification: Endophthalmitis can be of several types:**

a)  Sterile Endophthalmitis : Also named as TASS or Toxic Anterior Segment Syndrome
b)  Acute Bacterial Infective Endophthalmitis
c)  Acute Fungal Infective Endophthalmitis
d)  Chronic Endophthalmitis
e)  Endogenous Endophthalmitis (metastatic Endophthalmitis)

## TOXIC ANTERIOR SEGMENT SYNDROME: TASS

Sterile Endophthalmitis also termed TASS, is a sterile inflammation that occurs after anterior segment surgery. It can occur sporadically or in clusters to several patients undergoing surgery on the same day. TASS tends to occur as a result of immune reaction from the patient's body to the materials used during surgery which is not infective in nature.

**The following is an incomplete list of causes of TASS :**

a) **Abnormal solutions, like denatured BSS**
b) **Contamination of equipment, and IOLs**
c) **Irrigation solutions (abnormal pH or ionic composition),**
d) **Denatured viscoelastic,**
e) **Residual detergent in reusable equipment**
f) **Chemical residues left after sterilization.**
g) **Residual lens cortex,**
h) **Preservatives in ophthalmic solutions, and**
i) **Endotoxins that is not destroyed by the sterilization process**

**Clinical Presentation:**

**TASS** presents as severe intraocular inflammation within 24 to 48 hours after surgery.

It is always negative for Gram stain and no causative organism can be found. Clinical symptoms include:

1) Mild to moderate Pain and conjunctival injection
2) Blurred vision and reduced Visual acuity.
3) Acute Flare and cells in the anterior chamber.
4) Hypopyon with Fibrinous exudates in the A/C
5) Mild to severe corneal edema
6) Dilated Pupil which is sluggish or non reacting to light
7) IOP may be increased

The most important factor is the time of onset; TASS usually starts within 24 hours postoperatively. More delayed onset 2-7 days have been reported, but it is most common to start within 24 to 48 hours of surgery. Most of the Infective Endophthalmitis usually starts after 24 hours, therefore, any Endophthalmitis presenting on the first post operative day should raise the suspicion of TASS.

Second important factor is that the inflammation is mainly confined in the anterior segment with very little inflammation of the vitreous. Therefore, on B scan if the vitreous is clear, it may be an indicator that the condition is not infective in nature. In the case of infective Endophthalmitis, the vitreous is often involved and vitreous opacity is present.

On Gram stain and culture of the aqueous and vitreous tap usually yields negative results. Severe pain, chemosis of the eyelids are present in infective Endophthalmitis, while TASS is less painful and not associated with lid edema. Cornel edema is more severe in TASS and less severe in Infective Endophthalmitis.

In fact the factors responsible for excessive inflammation and TASS are very diverse and are difficult to identify in all cases. The surgeon has to take into consideration of all the materials and instruments that enters the eye during surgery or immediately after the surgery that may cause inflammatory response and damage through toxicity to the etiologic agents.

## MANAGEMENT:

Before treatment is started, infective Endophthalmitis has to be excluded.

**Grading : Sterile Endophthalmitis may be graded according to severity.**

Grade 1 : No Corneal edema, protracted inflammation present no hypopyon, Visual acuity better than 6/18

Grade 2 : Corneal edema present but not severe. Early hypopyon, pupil reacting to light Visual acuity worse than 6/60

Grade 3 : Profound Corneal edema often Limbus to Limbus, big Hypopyon Fibrinous exudates in anterior chamber and Pupil Dilated, Visual acuity drops to perception of light.

## TREATMENT OF TASS:

Treatment may be started according to severity. Topical steroids are the treatment of choice in grade 1 disease. Initially, Prednesolone Acetate 1% eye drops hourly or two hourly is started. Topical antibiotics like Moxifloxacin has no role in TASS, but should be prescribed to avoid secondary infection. Topical cycloplegics and NSAID drops may be required if there is pain.

In more severe cases, at Stage 2 and 3, Sub- Tenon's injection of soluble Steroid like Dexamethasone and Depo -steroid, either Depo Medrol or Triamcinolone acetonide is given. This is supported by topical steroid drops. Systemic steroid 80 mg Prednesolone immediately and tapered as the inflammation reduces.

Stronger cycloplegics such as Homatropine 2% or Atropine 1% eye drops is added to break pupillary block due to inflammatory membrane. If the Intraocular pressure is high, oral agents like Acetazolamide and topical beta blocker drops are added to reduce IOP.

The patients should be followed closely, especially if there is any question of an infectious etiology. Inflammation secondary to TASS will respond readily to steroid treatment, which may then be tapered accordingly. These patients may also have concomitant Trabecular meshwork damage and IOP must be monitored closely during the recovery period.

Should a case of TASS be detected, this must be taken seriously by all the staff that handles the equipments and safety procedures reviewed. It should be borne in mind that, Endophthalmitis, whether sterile or infectious, is a serious and potentially devastating complication of cataract surgery and must be avoided by all means. This requires concerted efforts of all the staff working in the hospital to make it possible.

## INFECTIVE ENDOPHTHALMITIS:

**Infective endophthalmitis** may be bacterial, fungal or mixed infection. It is very difficult to distinguish between the Infective and sterile endophthalmitis. TASS usually presents in the first 24 hours after surgery and infectious endophthalmitis usually presents later. Bacterial Endophthalmitis presents 24 to 48 hours after surgery. Fungal endophthalmitis presents later may be week or month after surgery. Sterile and infectious endophthalmitis can have overlap in clinical presentation rendering it difficult to diagnose. Very low virulent organisms may cause chronic endophthalmitis presenting months after surgery.

**The most common presenting signs and symptoms of infectious endophthalmitis are:**

a) Pain usually moderate to severe, however some cases may pay present with little pain

b) Decreased or blurred vision,

c) Lid swelling and chemosis rendering the lids to close,

d) Protracted conjunctival injection and chemosis,

e) Mild Corneal Edema

f) There is an increased cellular reaction in the anterior chamber, but not Fibrinous.

g) Hypopyon seen upon presentation in majority of patients.

h) Unusual presentations include retinal vasculitis, and mid-peripheral retinal hemorrhages

**Etiologic agents involved in infective endophthalmitis:**

1. **Bacterial postoperative acute endophthalmitis:**
   a. **Acute endophthalmitis:**
      (1)    Staphylococcus epidermidis.
      (2)    Staphylococcus aureus.
      (3)    Streptococcus
      (4)    Gram-negative species:
      (a)    Pseudomonas.
      (b)    Proteus.
      (c)    Escherichia coli.

   b. **Chronic low grade: Bacterial Post operative endophthalmitis:**
      (1)    Staphylococcus epidermidis.
      (2)    Propionibacterium acnes.

2. **Endogenous Bacterial endophthalmitis:**
   a.    Streptococcus sp. (pneumococcus, viridens).
   b.    Staph. aureus

3. **Post Filter bleb Bacterial endophthalmitis**
   a.    Haemophilus influenzae.
   b.    Streptococcus sp.

4. **Fungal—postoperative**
   a. Volutella.
   b. Neurospora.
   c. Fusarium.
   d. Candida.

6. **Fungal Endogenous :** Candida.
7. **Fungal Traumatic** : Fusarium and Aspergillus

**The clinical manifestations of endophthalmitis may sometimes be used to**

**Differentiate between bacterial, fungal, and sterile etiologic agents. These manifestations**

**are as follows:**

1. **Sterile Endophthalmitis :**
   a. Presents early usually within first 24 hours after surgery.
   b. Little or moderate pain
   c. Fibrinous Exudates and rarely hypopyon
   d. No Lid edema and moderate congestion

2. **Bacterial**
   a. Sudden onset (1 to 7 days postoperatively), rapid progression.
   b. Severe Pain, very red, chemosis of the conjunctiva.
   c. Lid edema and spasm.
   d. Rapid loss of vision.
   e. Hypopyon and vitreous involvement.

3. **Fungal or low-grade bacterial**
   a. Delayed onset (8 to 14 days or more).
   b. Some pain and redness.
   c. Transient hypopyon.
   d. Localized anterior vitreous gray-white patch.
   e. Satellite lesions.
   f. Vision reduced to light perception.
   g. Rarely, severe exudation into anterior chamber.

**Preoperative risk factors for infectious endophthalmitis are:**

a)  Blepharitis,

b)  Conjunctivitis,

c)  Canaliculitis,

d)  Lachrymal duct obstruction,

e)  Contact lens wear,

f)  Ocular prosthesis in the fellow orbit.

g)  Implantation of a secondary intraocular lens (IOL) increases the incidence of endophthalmitis,

h)  Diabetes Malitus,

i)  Trans-scleral suture fixation IOL

Intraocular bacterial contamination is the primary cause of infectious endophthalmitis resulting from inadequate eye lid preparation.

## TREATMENT OF ENDOPHTHALMITIS:

Endophthalmitis, whether sterile or infectious, is a serious and potentially sight threatening complication of cataract surgery. The condition is an ocular emergency and immediate hospitalization is recommended. If the endophthalmitis presents within 24 hours after surgery, this should be treated as TASS with steroids and other protocols.

If the condition presents 24 hours after surgery, this should be treated as bacterial Endophthalmitis until and unless proven otherwise. Standard treatment for infectious endophthalmitis includes intravitreal antibiotics, with or without pars plana vitrectomy, topical and subconjunctival antibiotics, and corticosteroid therapy. If no clinical improvement is noted within the first 48 to 72 hours, vitreous tap and intravitreal antibiotic injection should be repeated, and pars plana vitrectomy performed.

## IDENTIFICATION OF PATHOGEN:

Samples for culture should be obtained from aqueous and vitreous to confirm the diagnosis. It is to be borne in mind that, negative culture does not rule out infection.

**Procedure to collect samples from Aqueous:**

a) Povidone-iodine 5% is instilled and the eye is draped. The eye is washed with BSS

b) Anaesthesia : Topical and subconjunctival or peribulbar injection anaesthesia is administered.

**Collection of Aqueous samples**

a) 0.1-0.2ml of aqueous is aspirated via a limbal paracentesis using a 25 G needle on a tuberculin syringe.

**b) The syringe is capped and labeled and sent to the laboratory**

**Collection of vitreous samples:**

a) A 2ml syringe and a 23G needle may be used to collect a vitreous sample.

b) A special disposable vitrector may be used to collect vitreous sample.

c) The distance from the limbus for the scleral puncture is measured with calipers and marked 4mm (in pseudophakic eye) or 3mm (in aphakic eye).

d) The needle or vitrector is introduced and a vitreous sample 0.2 to 0.4ml are aspirated from the mid-vitreous cavity

## TREATMENT

A. **Intravitreal antibiotics** are the main tools in the management of Bacterial Endophthalmitis. The intravitreal injection antibiotics achieve levels above the minimum inhibitory concentration of most pathogens. Intravitreal injections should be carried out immediately after culture specimens have been obtained without waiting for the culture and sensitivity report. Depending upon the severity of inflammation, the following antibiotics are commonly given:

- If gram positive organism is suspected, vancomycin 1 mg in 0.1 ml is injected.
- If gram negative organism is suspected, ceftazidime 2.25 mg/0.1 mL is given
- If mixed etiology is suspected, both the drugs are given as intravitreal injection
- Other antibiotics are given if the culture report shows specific sensitivity.

B. **Periocular antibiotic injections:**

In addition to the intravitreal injection, periocular or sub conjunctival injections are also used but of doubtful additional benefit. Injection of vancomycin 50mg and ceftazidime 125mg (or amikacin 50mg) given separately in the periocular region after topical anesthesia. Gentamycin 40 mg / ml: 1/2 ml (20 mg in 0.5 ml) subconjunctival injection is also preferred.

C. **Topical antibiotics** are of limited benefit, Fortified Gentamycin and Vancomycin may be applied frequently and may reach therapeutic levels in the anterior chamber.

D. **Topical Cycloplegics**: Homatropine or Atropine eye drops for cycloplegia every two hours until pupil dilatation is obtained and three time daily thereafter.

E. **Oral antibiotics** Fluoroquinolones penetrate the eye and moxifloxacin 400mg daily for 10 days is recommended; Clarithromycin 500mg bid. may be helpful for culture-negative infections.

F. **Oral steroids.** The rationale for the use of steroids is to limit the destructive complications of the inflammatory process. Oral Prednisolone 60mg daily should be started in severe cases 24 hours after intravitreal antibiotics injection is given provided that, fungal infection has been excluded by examination of smears.

G. **Periocular steroids** dexamethasone (12mg) or triamcinolone (1.0mg) should be considered if systemic therapy is contraindicated.

H. **Topical dexamethasone** 0.1% q.i.d to treat anterior uveitis.

I. **Intravitreal steroids** is controversial. It reduces inflammation in the short term it does not influence the final visual result. Intravitreal Injection of steroids may be avoided to minimize toxic effect on retina.

J. **Pars Plana Vitrectomy**:

Pars plana vitrectomy is performed on patients who have unsatisfactory response to the initial treatment. The results of the EVS study group on a large series of patients since 1995 show positive benefit of Vitrectomy on patients presenting with perception of light. It is also documented that, diabetic patients benefit from vitrectomy irrespective of presentation.

Vitrectomy is beneficial because it removes all vitreous membranes, debris, and the infecting organisms and associated toxins.

**Aqueous sample and vitreous sample should be sent to the laboratory for :**

a) **Gram Stain, Giemsa stain and Calcofluor stain and result immediately obtained.**

b) **Bacterial Culture inoculation in sheep blood agar plate, chocolate agar plate, beef heart infusion, thioglycolate broth and is incubated at 37 degrees C for 36 to 72hours.**

c) **Fungal Culture should be placed in Sabouraud medium and blood agar plate and incubated at 30 degree C for 36 to 72 hours**

d) **Polymerase Chain Reaction (PCR) can be useful to identify unusual organisms.**

**Further management of Bacterial endophthalmitis:**

After the initial treatment is started based on the diagnosis from presentation, examination of smear and culture results, ultrasound B scan is helpful to assess the response to treatment.

A. Signs of improvement: If there are signs of improvement and culture report is obtained which do not dictate change of antibiotic therapy, the same treatment is continued.

B. In case a different antibiotic is shown to be sensitive, subconjunctival injection and topical treatment is modified further intravitreal injection is not indicated if there is signs of improvement.

C. In case the signs are getting worse after 48 hours and the organism is found to be sensitive to a different antibiotic, Vitrectomy and intravitreal injection of the antibiotic to which the organisms are sensitive is given.

D. Prognosis depends upon the virulence of the organisms involved and the duration of presentation before the treatment is started.

## PREPARATION OF ANTIBIOTICS FOR INTRAVIREAL INJECTION:

A. **Ceftazidime Hydrochloride: Dose: 2.25 mg in 0.1 ml/ Cefazolin sodium: 2.25 mg in 0.1 ml**
   - **Commercially available in 250 mg, 500 mg and 1 G dry powder in vial**
   - Add 10 ml of diluents (0.9 % Sodium Chloride or Distilled Water) to 500 mg powder in vial or, 5 ml diluents to 250 mg powder in vial.
   - Now you have 50 mg/ml concentration.
   - Take 1 ml (50 mg) and add 1.2 ml diluents(0.9 % Sodium chloride) resultant solution of 2.2 ml has 22.72 mg/ ml

   **Withdraw 0.1 ml containing 2.272 mg in tuberculin syringe : Ready for Injection**

B. **Vancomycin Dose : 1 mg /0.1 ml :**

**Preparation : The vial contains 500 mg powder : Check the vial for presentation which may contain 500 mg in vial, 1G vial or 5 mg/ml in 10 ml Syringe for pediatric use.**

- Add 10 ml of distilled water to 500 mg powder in vial.

- Now 1 ml contains 50 mg: concentration 50 mg/ml.

- Take 2 ml or 100 mg and add 8 ml distilled water in 10 ml syringe :

- The resulting solution 10 ml contains 100 mg that is, the solution contains 10 mg/ml.

- **Withdraw 0.1 ml in a tuberculin syringe: Now you have 1 mg in 0.1 ml solution : Ready for Injection.**

- **If other concentration in vial is used, dilute appropriate concentration to reach 1mg/0.1 ml**

**C. Amikacin : Dose 0.2 to 0.4 mg in 0.1 ml**

- One vial contains 500 mg in 2 ml (250 mg/ml) solution.

- Take 0.8 ml solution and mix with 9.2 ml of diluents to give total 10 ml

- Now the solution has a concentration of 200 mg in 10 ml (20mg/ml).

- From 20 mg /ml solution withdraw 0.2 ml (4 mg) and mix with 0.8 ml of diluents in a second syringe to achieve final solution of 4 mg / ml

- **Take 0.1 ml in a tuberculin syringe. Now 0.1 ml contain 0.4 mg ready for injection.**

- **For concentration 0.2 mg in 0.1 ml, half of the dose is to be diluted :**

- **From 20mg/ml solution take 0.1 ml : 2 mg and add 0.9 ml diluant. Now 1 ml contains 2 mg.**

- **Withdraw 0.1 ml in tuberculin syringe containing 0.2 mg/01 ml : ready for injection**

**D. Gentamycin sulfate: Dose 0.1 to 0.2 mg in 0.1 ml (Rarely used due to retinal toxicity)**

- One vial contains 80 mg in 2 ml (40 mg/ml) solution.

- Take 0.1 ml (4 mg) solution into a disposable syringe, and mix with 3.9 ml of diluant. Now you have a solution of 4 mg in 4 ml or 1 mg/1 ml

- **Take 0.1 ml which has 0.1 mg /0.1 ml : Ready for injection**

E. **Clindamycin phosphate: Dose 1 mg in 0.1 ml (Rarely used because of Retina Toxicity)**

- One Vial contains a 600 mg in 4 ml solution (150 mg/1 ml)
- Take 0.2 ml (30 mg) solution into a syringe and mix with 2.8 ml of distilled water to get a solution of 3 ml containing 30 mg or 10 mg / ml
- **Take 0.1 ml in tuberculin syringe 1 mg/0.1 ml: ready for injection.**

Gentamycin and Clindamycin are retinotoxic and should only be used when better alternatives do not exist.

For preparation of intravitreal antibiotics, sterility must be maintained, the diluents used should be either pure distilled sterile water or 0.9 % sodium chloride solution. For all medications, the volume from the final solution for intravitreal injection is 0.1 ml drawn into a tuberculin syringe and injection given separately. If multiple drugs are to be injected, the needle is kept in place and the syringe is changed.

## FUNGAL ENDOPHTHALMITIS:

Fungal endophthalmitis presents one week after the surgical procedure and presents with mild pain and redness, turbid vitreous less anterior chamber reaction, satellite lesions, and transient Hypopyon. If suspected, immediate vitrectomy, culture and gram staining of the aspirate and intravitreal injection of amphotrecin B is the first choice of treatment.

The following management is suggested:

1. **Vitrectomy is performed immediately**
2. Intravitreal injection of Amphotrecin B
3. Oral Amphotrecin B
4. Topical Natamycin or Amphotrecin B hourly.
5. Ketoconazole is antagonistic to Amphotrecin B and should not be used together.
6. Cycloplegic eye drops 2 hourly
7. Antibiotic eye drops to prevent secondary infection.

## PREPARATION OF INTRAVITREAL AMPHOTRECIN B:
**Dose : Amphotrecin B: 0.005 mg in 0.1 ml**
- Commercial vial contains 50 mg powder.

- Add 10 ml of diluent to reconstitute the 50 mg powder
- Now the solution contains a concentration of 5 mg/ml.
- Add 0.1 ml (0.5 mg) of reconstituted solution with 9.9 ml of distilled water.
- Total 10 ml now contain 0.5 mg
- Now 1 ml contain 0.05 mg.
- Final solution of 0.05 mg/ 1ml. or 0.005 mg in 0.1 ml
- **Take 0.1 ml in tuberculin syringe : Ready for injection**

**Systemic Antifungal :**

a) **Amphotrecin B :** 1 mg in 500 ml saline slow IV over 4 hours as test dose. Then increase to 5-10 mg / day slow IV

b) **Fluconazole :** 400 to 800 mg Oral / day

c) **Ketoconazole :** 200 to 400 mg Oral / bid and stop Amhotercin B.

## SUMMARY OF MANAGEMENT OF POST OPERATIVE ENDOPHTHALMITIS:

Post Operative endophthalmitis whether sterile or infective is a dangerous complication. The surgeon may become horror stricken so that the normal judgment response may be dull and difficult for the surgeon to decide what to do and what to say to the patient and to the relatives. This may cause unnecessary delay in diagnosis and treatment resulting in much worse prognosis.

The correct way to deal with the situation is to explain to the relatives the situation, hospitalize the patient and initiate treatment as soon as possible. My advice is to consult a vitreo-retina specialist right from the beginning. A clear plan of management is discussed between the doctors and started immediately. **The following are some suggestions for a plan of management of endophthalmitis:**

1. If the condition presents next day after surgery, treat as Sterile Endophthalmitis. After hospitalization, Aqueous Tap and vitreous tap is performed and samples sent for gram stain and culture. Topical and Sub Tenon Steroid is immediately given along with cycloplegics and broad spectrum antibiotics. The preferred topical steroids are Prednisolone acetate 1% and Dexamethasone 0.1 % eye drops. The recommended oral steroid is prednisone is 30 mg to 60 mg per day for 5 to 10days and then tapered. Intravitreal Steroid is reserved for giving at the time of vitrectomy if required. It is better to wait until Gram Stain report is obtained before intravitreal Steroid is given. The gram stain can be done very quickly by the laboratory staff. By the time full laboratory results are obtained, the

condition improves and vision usually becomes better in a case of TASS. Most of the sterile endophthalmitis if appropriately treated a regains vision 6/12 or better.

2. **If after described Steroid therapy for TASS the condition does not improve within 24 hours, and if the inflammation increases or hypopyon increases, this should be treated as bacterial endophthalmitis and intravitreal antibiotic injection should be given immediately.**

3. If the patient presents with endophthalmitis any time after 48 hours of surgery, this is treated as Acute Bacterial Endophthalmitis. Aqueous and vitreous tap is performed and Intravitreal injection of Vancomycin and Ceftazidime is immediately given and hourly Fortified Gentamycin and vancomycin topical eye drops is started with Cycloplegic and systemic IV Ceftriaxone or Amikacin 15 mg per kg body weight immediately. Wait for laboratory reports and closely monitor the patient for improvement. If no improvement is noted in 48 hours, the reports are reviewed and the patient is sent for vitrectomy.

4. If the patient presents with visual acuity perception of light and severe inflammation, send for immediate vitrectomy and send the samples for laboratory investigations including culture and sensitivity. Usual treatment for acute bacterial endophthalmitis is to be followed.

5. If the patient presents at any time between 7 to 14 days after surgery, treat this as Fungal Endophthalmitis and perform immediate vitrectomy and treat in the line of fungal infection.

6. Late post operative endophthalmitis due to low virulent bacteria is possible. This is to be treated according to the prescribed guidelines.

Never get a panic attack if endophthalmitis is encountered. A high volume surgeon must confront with some cases of endophthalmitis during the clinical life. Explanation to the patient and to the relatives is very difficult. My usual way to explain is, the patient has developed an unusual type of inflammation for which an urgent and intensive care is required. The patient needs to be hospitalized for intensive nursing and surgical care, and we will do all our best so that the patient can recover from the complication as soon as possible. We will also call other Ophthalmologists for consultation and appropriate intervention should that becomes necessary. In my experience, this is all that required to convince the patient and the relatives to accept the situation. If appropriately treated, you will get good outcome in all cases of sterile endophthalmitis and most of the Bacterial endophthalmitis cases. Worst prognosis is for the Fungal endophthalmitis but fortunately is not a common condition.

## Delayed-onset postoperative endophthalmitis

Delayed-onset endophthalmitis develops following cataract surgery when an organism of low virulence infects the eye during surgery. The infection may be caused by *P. acnes* and

S. epidermidis, Corynebacterium spp. or Candida specis

The onset of presentation ranges from 4 weeks to 9 months postoperatively and typically follows uneventful surgery.

It may also be followed by YAG-laser capsulotomy when the organisms are confined in the anterior chamber before the YAG laser is done. The organisms gain access to the vitreous through the Yag Laser posterior capsular gap and cause posterior segment involvement and inflammation.

**The patient presents with** painless mild progressive visual loss and may complain of floaters.

**Signs and symptoms:**

1) Low-grade anterior uveitis, with mild cells and flare
2) Mutton-fat keratic precipitates (KP)may be present
3) Inflammation of the vitreous rarely Hypopyon may be present.
4) Blurring of vision which is unstable and fluctuates.

### 3. Investigations.
The diagnosis should be confirmed by cultures of the aqueous and vitreous tap with growth and identification of the organism.

Anaerobic culture should be performed if P. *acnes* infection is suspected
Detection rate of pathogens can be greatly improved with PCR.

## 4. Clinical course.

Without antibiotic treatment the inflammation responds well to topical steroids and recurs when steroid treatment is stopped and eventually becomes chronic in nature.

## 5. Treatment:

**Intravitreal vancomycin** (1mg in 0.1ml) is the antibiotic of choice.

According to the sensitivity, methicillin, cefazolin and clindamycin may also be given when report is available. Try to avoid clindamycin because of possible retinal toxicity.

**6. Vitrectomy with removal of IOL** may be required in resistant cases. After the initial treatment, if good aphakia is obtained and vision is preserved, secondary sulcus fixated IOL may be implanted as a secondary procedure.

## PREVENTION OF ENDOPHTHALMITIS:

**It is prudent for the ophthalmologist to try to avoid endophthalmitis by all means.**

Surgical conditions vary in different circumstances with different surgeons. It is not possible to describe a set of uniform procedures to prevent all endophthalmitis. I shall discuss the common procedures to avoid endophthalmitis but shall recommend that the individual surgeons formulate his or her own protocol to avoid endophthalmitis.

I have performed surgeries under different settings, eye camp in open school class rooms, controlled operation theaters, Eye Operation theaters in General Hospitals, contaminated general surgery operation theaters, indigenous clinic where normal room is converted to eye Operation Theater. At every situation I have prepared my own protocol to avoid endophthalmitis particular to that circumstance. I have also reviewed the protocol of advanced centers in USA and UK.

## PREVENTION OF STERILE ENDOPHTHALMITIS

It is most difficult to prevent sterile endophthalmitis because all substances that are used during the surgery may cause protracted inflammation in spite of the fact that meticulous measures has been taken to prevent infection. The surgeon needs to be careful about each and every material and instrument introduced into the anterior chamber.

The most important step in preventing toxic anterior segment syndrome (TASS) is to minimize the possibility of contamination with potentially toxic substances, including and substance that may be attached to the instruments.

1. First, the cleaning and sterilization process can be periodically reviewed to avoid unwanted residues left on equipment.

2. All instruments must be carefully cleaned and dried prior to placing them in the autoclave.

3. Hot air oven require special mention because, instruments must be cleaned and fully dried before placing in hot air oven. Residues of previous surgery remaining on the instruments may dry up and be introduced into the eye during subsequent surgery. These substances contain denatured protein residues of previous patient and may cause sterile inflammation.

4. If reusable tubing are used it must be cleaned, flushed and dried before placing in the autoclave and allowed to cool after taking out of the autoclave.

5. Disposable tubing is ideal to avoid contamination with residues from previous surgeries.

6. Viscoelastic cannulas, irrigation and aspiration cannulas and phaco tips require meticulous cleaning and flushing with BSS and also dried. I found a hair drier handy for drying the instruments.

7. If ultrasound cleaner is used, the distilled water must be replaced at every cycle.

8. Phacoemulsification machines can be periodically checked for back flush or other sources for contamination.

9. Solutions used during surgery can also be sources of toxicity.

10. Any drops placed in the conjunctival sac containing preservatives and betadine iodine must be washed out before commencing the surgery. Any remnants of these substances gaining access into the anterior chamber during surgery may cause protracted inflammation.

11. Balanced salt solution should be at room temperature or cold but fresh bottle for each case should be used. If multiple surgeries are performed from one bottle of BSS, the infusion set should be discarded after each surgery and a new infusion set is used every time.

12. Denatured viscoelastic must be avoided and have a good supply of Viscoelastics: Never re- use viscoelastic, but if you want to do so, be careful to keep the syringe sterile and change the Cannula by replacing it with a fresh sterile one. Don't expose the Intraocular Lens to operation room atmospheric air for a long period of time by opening the packet long before insertion.

13. The knives, cannulas and lens injector cartridge should be washed with fresh sterile BSS before introducing into the anterior chamber.

14. Last but not the least, surgeon's hands and gloves must be washed before surgery with BSS to remove all powder and sterile but contaminating materials.

In case endophthalmitis is detected in any post operative patient, this must be taken seriously by all the staff members that handle the equipments and instruments. The safety procedures are to be reviewed. It should be borne in mind that, Endophthalmitis, whether sterile or infectious is a devastating complication of cataract surgery and must be avoided by all means. This requires concerted efforts of all the staff working in the hospital to make it possible.

**Prevention of bacterial and fungal Endophthalmitis: A very comprehensive guideline is discussed at the article of ESCRS please refer for the full article ESCRS Guidelines on *prevention*, investigation and management of post-operative Endophthalmitis Version 2. August 2007. Editors. Peter Barry, Wolfgang**

It is the size of inoculation of the bacterial load that causes bacterial endophthalmitis. The sources of contamination should be critically examined and prevented.

The main sources of bacteria are:

1.  Operation room air
2.  Operation table and floor.
3.  Patient's own bacteria from lids and conjunctival sac and clothing.
4.  Instruments containing bacteria from previous surgery specially if reused.
5.  Contaminated Irrigating fluid and viscoelastics
6.  Surgeons and assistants hands and mouth.
7.  Fellow patients when multiple surgeries are performed on a single day.

## GENERAL GUIDELINES TO PREVENT INFECTIVE ENDOPHTHALMITIS

1.  On the day of surgery, and every day the floor and the operation table and microscope body must be cleaned with disinfectants. This must include all horizontal surfaces including the floor.
2.  OR air is cleaned with laminar flow and Hepa Filters.
3.  In indigenous operation theatres, Fumigation with Formalin twice a week and using disinfectant air spray in the morning will keep the air reasonably germ free and clean.
4.  Ultraviolet Tube Light kept on all night before surgery is another preventive measure for the operation room air.
5.  Patients clothing should be exchanged outside the operation room and an autoclaved patient dress should be given to each patient.
6.  The eye and face of the patient should be cleaned with bactericidal soap in the waiting area. Treat any Blepharitis and dacryocystitis prior to cataract surgery.

7.  Broad spectrum antibiotics like ciprofloxacin eye drops 48 hours before surgery and in the morning of surgery at least three times.

8.  Apply one drop Povidone Iodine 5 % in the conjunctival sac in the preparation room.

9.  Apply 10 % povidone iodine to the skin around the eye as skin asepsis.

10. Wash hands with antiseptic soap and povidone iodine and chlorhexidine

11. Apply drapes and confine the eye lashes from the surgical field under the drapes.

12. Perform Phacoemulsification or SICS surgery as planned.

13. Clean and wash each instrument with sterile BSS before introducing into the eye

14. Put one drop of Povidone iodine 5% and one drop of antibiotic drop in the conjunctival sac at the end of surgery.

15. Subconjunctival antibiotic is not advocated, and is optional. If complications like PCR, vitreous loss has happened, intracameral vancomycin or cefuroxime and sub conjunctival gentamycin may be given.

16. Each person in the Operation area must have a defined job description and must know exactly what he or she is expected to do within the surgical area.

17. The instrument cleaning should not be kept waiting until the end of surgery day and should be cleaned as soon as one surgery is complete. Waiting for long period results in drying of blood and other materials on the instrument and cannot be removed later on. When this passes through the Hot air oven, sterile altered protein and other inflammatory materials stick to the instruments.

18. Autoclave every instrument to be used during surgery and nothing should go inside the eye which is not freshly Autoclaved or otherwise sterilized. Hot air Oven is also very good for sterilizing the instruments in between surgeries. If you have multiple surgeries in a single day, use separate sets of instruments, Phaco Tips, knives, Cannulas each one sterilized just prior to the surgery. It is actually very easy to do so. You need only Three Sets of instruments. Use one set for the surgery you are performing, one set for the Next Case and Put the Other set in the Autoclave or Hot air oven. By the time you finish the first surgery, the third set will be sterilized for the next surgery. It does not cost much to have three Sets of instruments, because we use very limited number of instruments to perform Cataract Surgery and in the present day situation, you can actually perform good SICS or Phaco surgery only with Eight Instruments.

19. Train your Assistants to help you at every step of the surgery; they must know what you expect them to do. Talking may increase the spread of organisms from droplets discharged during talking. In my surgery, I never have to say a word while performing the surgery. The assistant must know how to put drops on the cornea, when to mop up excess fluid if necessary, and hand over each piece of instrument at every step you do. Here again

repeated practice by yourself and the assistant is required. They must be able to help you at every step during surgery or complications thereof. Once you train your assistants, you will find that Cataract Surgery, Phaco, SICS or ECCE is not difficult at all. After some time you will find that cataract surgery is the most rewarding surgery, because with an effort of 15 minutes, you can restore sight to a blind person.

20. If operating at an indigenous general surgery operation theatre where a dedicated Ophthalmic Operation Room is not available, it is very difficult to prevent endophthalmitis. Sterile air obtained by drawing air into an empty 2 cc syringe inside the sterile package is introduced into the anterior chamber at the end of surgery to replace the potentially infected BSS in the A/C. Ocular surface is washed with BSS mixed with antibiotics, one drop Povidone Iodine 5% and antibiotic eye drops at the end of surgery may be useful to prevent infection. This reduces the bacterial load and hopefully will prevent endophthalmitis.

**This is to be remembered that, an all out concerted effort of all the Operation Room personnel is required to prevent Endophthalmitis.**

## REFERENCES :

1. ESCRS Guidelines on *prevention*, investigation and management of post-operative *endophthalmitis*. Version 2. August 2007. Editors. Peter Barry, Wolfgang

2. Aaberg TM, Flynn HW, Schiffman J, et al. Nosocomial acute-onset postoperative endophthalmitis survey. Ophthalmology. 1998;105:1004-1010.

3. Donnenfeld ED, Perry HD. Cataract surgery: five ways to prevent endophthalmitis. Rev Ophthalmol. 1996;3:67-72.

4. Ormerod LD, Ho DD, Becker LE, et al. Endophthalmitis caused by coagulase-negative staphylococci. Ophthalmology. 1993;100:715-723.

5. Endophthalmitis Vitrectomy Study Group: Results of the endophthalmitis vitrectomy study: a randomized trial of immediate vitrectomy and of intravenous antibiotics for the treatment of postoperative bacterial endophthalmitis. Arch Ophthalmol. 1995;113:1479-1496

6. Godley BF, Folk JC. Retinal hemorrhages as an early sign of acute bacterial endophthalmitis. Am J Ophthalmol. 1993;116:247-249.

7. Dickey JB, Thompson KD, Jay WN. Anterior chamber aspirate cultures after uncomplicated cataract surgery. Am J Ophthalmol. 1991;112:278-282

8. Doft BH, Wisniewski SR, Kelsey SF, et al. Diabetes and postoperative endophthalmitis in the endophthalmitis vitrectomy study. Arch Ophthalmol. 2001;119:650-656.

9. Endophthalmitis Vitrectomy Study Group. Microbiologic factors and visual outcomes in the endophthalmitis vitrectomy study. Am J Ophthalmol. 1996;122:830-846.

10. Speaker MG, Milch FA, Shaf MK, et al. Role of external bacterial flora and the pathogenesis of acute postoperative endophthalmitis. Ophthalmology. 1991;98:639-649.

11. Montan PG, Koranyi G, Setterquist HE, et al. Endophthalmitis after cataract surgery: risk factors relating to technique and events of the operation and patient history. Ophthalmology. 1998;105:1271-1277.

12. Nelson DB, Donnenfeld ED, Perry HD. Sterile endophthalmitis after sutureless cataract surgery. Ophthalmology. 1992;99:1655-1657.

13. Doft BH, Kelsey SF, Wisniewski SR. Additional procedures after the initial vitrectomy or tap-biopsy in the endophthalmitis vitrectomy study. Ophthalmology. 1998;105:707-716.

14. Haider SA, Hassett P, Bron AJ. Intraocular vancomycin levels after intravitreal injection in post cataract extraction endophthalmitis. Retina. 2001;21:210-213.

15. Irvine DW, Flynn HW, Miller D, et al. Endophthalmitis caused by gram-negative organisms. Arch Ophthalmol. 1992;110:1450-1454.

16. Sternberg P, Martin D. Management of endophthalmitis in the post-endophthalmitis vitrectomy study era. Arch Ophthalmol. 2001;119:254-255.

17. Liesegang TJ. Use of antimicrobials to prevent postoperative infection in patients with cataracts. Curr Opin Ophthalmol. 2001;12:68-74.

18. Shah G, Stein J, Sharma S, et al. Visual outcomes following the use of intravitreal steroids in the treatment of postoperative endophthalmitis. Ophthalmology. 2000;107:486-489.

# Chapter 19
# POST OPERATIVE CME

CME is due to development of fluid filled (cystoid) spaces in the outer plexiform layer and the inner nuclear layer of the retina. The term is cystoid and not cystic because the fluid-filled spaces are not true cyst. Many cases of CME are subclinical and detected only on fluorescein angiography. In clinically significant cases, patients may complain of decreased vision or of visual distortion. Clinically-significant CME in post-cataract extraction cases often manifests as visual decline to 20/40 or worse.

**Causes :**

The following diseases may cause CME,

a) Diabetic retinopathy,
b) Venous occlusive disease,
c) Hypertension,
d) Choroidal neovascularization,
e) Retinal vascular malformations, tumors, radiation retinopathy,
f) Uveitis, epiretinal membranes, retinitis pigmentosa
g) Intraocular surgery including Cataract Surgery.

## POST OPERATIVE CME :

Postoperative CME, is also known as Irvine-Gass Syndrome. This was originally described by Irvine in 1953, and fluorescein angiographic changes of CME was described by Gass and Norton in 1966. Clinically significant CME generally occurs within 4 to 12 weeks after surgery. The incidence of postoperative CME varies between 5% to 15% after Intracapsular cataract extraction. Studies using fluorescein angiography demonstrated an overall incidence of 36% to 60% following intracapsular cataract extraction. Incidence of angiographically evident CME following Extracapsular cataract extraction is between 10 % to 15 %.

The incidence of CME increases with capsular rupture, and adherence of vitreous to the surgical wound. Early YAG LASER posterior capsulotomy may increase the incidence of CME.

**Mechanism of formation of CME:**

The exact mechanism of breakdown of the blood-retinal barrier and formation of Cystoid Macular Edema (CME) is not well understood. A number of theories have been discussed including Mechanical traction in the macular region by pull of vitreous, release of Prostaglandins due to inflammation and exposure to light or UV rays.

Several studies have been performed to understand the process of formation of CME and it now seems that, prostaglandin release contributes significantly in the development of CME and prostaglandin inhibitors are used both in prevention and treatment of the condition.

## CLINICAL PRESENTATION AND DIAGNOSIS:

Patients may be asymptomatic or may present with decreased visual acuity to 6/9 or 6/12 but may be as poor as 6/60. Patients also present with distortion of vision when examined by Amsler Grid, photophobia, ocular irritation, and floaters.

Pseudophakic CME should be suspected when a patient complains of decreased vision and distortion of Amsler grid following cataract extraction.

Clinically, retinal edema with cyst-like spaces in a honeycomb pattern around the fovea can be seen. On examination, visual acuity is reduced, the foveal reflex is dull and there may be signs of inflammation in the anterior chamber. The cystoid spaces may coalesce into a central larger space resulting in chronic edema and a lamellar hole can develop later.

Diagnosis is based on the typical clinical findings and characteristic appearance on fundus fluorescein angiography and OCT.

Angiographic CME is defined as cystoid macular edema that is not clinically noted by the physician or patient and is only detectable with fluorescein angiography.

The fluorescein angiogram gives a characteristic picture. Early phases of fluorescein angiography demonstrate dye leakage from the parafoveal retinal capillaries, and later phases of the angiogram demonstrate gradually increasing hyperfluorescence in a petaloid pattern around the fovea. The petaloid pattern of hyperfluorescence is characteristic of CME.

In late frames, staining of the optic disc is seen due to leakage of the peripapillary capillaries in Pseudophakic CME. In other common causes of CME such as diabetic macular edema, epiretinal fibrosis, and exudative macular degeneration, disc staining is not common.

## TREATMENT OF CME :

Several treatment modalities have been discussed in the treatment of Post operative Cystoid Macular Edema (CME):

1. **Topical Anti-inflammatories** : Nonsteroidal anti-inflammatory drugs (NSAID) such as ketorolac, diclofenac, flurbiprofen are cyclooxygenase inhibitors all block the conversion of arachidonic acid to prostaglandins. Topical NSAID (Xibrom) bromfenac sodium is said to have better penetration and have more benefit in the treatment of CME. Oral use of NSAID is of doubtful benefit but is often prescribed. Topical use of NSAID eye drops in the pre operative and post operative period especially in cases where are risk factors involved may reduce the incidence of CME.

2. **Corticosteroids:**
   Corticosteroids block the release of arachidonic acid from cell membranes and inhibit the formation of Prostaglandins. Topical and systemic Steroids have been shown to have potent anti inflammatory properties and may be beneficial in CME.

3. **Carbonic anhydrase inhibitors:** Acetazolamide (CAIs) stimulate the pumping action of the RPE, reducing the amount of fluid within the macula in CME. They have been demonstrated to be helpful in reducing CME in certain patients.

4. **Peribulbar Injection**: Subtenon's injections of Depo - Steroids theoretically deliver a higher dose of corticosteroids to the macula. There is a risk of prolonged elevation of intraocular pressure which must be monitored..

5. **Surgical Intervention**: In refractory cases, Nd. YAG laser vitreolysis, Vitrectomy and IOL removal have shown to be beneficial to resolve CME.

## Management Plan:

Post operative CME is a troublesome complication for the physician and the patient. No cause can be found and it reduces post operative visual acuity and is disappointing to the patient. Should this complication occur, a clear treatment plan should be in the mind of the surgeon:

1. Examine the patient with Three Mirror and Indirect Ophthalmoscopy
2. Perform a Fluorescein angiogram and OCT scan if available.
3. Prednesolone acetate 1% eye drops four times daily and bromfenac sodium eye drops two times daily for 4 weeks and monitor improvement.
4. Sub Tenon Injection Depo steroid half cc and dexamethasone half cc if IOP is not increased by previous use of topical steroids.
5. Oral Corticosteroids is indicated only if CME is complicated by inflammation and other risk factors like PCR and vitreous is in anterior chamber.
6. If condition is not improved within four weeks, consider vitrectomy.
7. Even after full resolution, the CME may recur and patients will complain of reduced color sensitivity and some visual disturbances especially in contrast sensitivity after the condition is resolved.

## Photo sensitization of Macula by Microscope light:

Much has been discussed about induced retinal injury by the use of the surgical microscope and this varies considerably among ophthalmologists. Retinal lesions caused by the operating microscope light are often found in the lower part of the macula. This may be a cause of delayed recovery of post operative vision, however it is found to resolve in few weeks after surgery.

Prevention of retinal toxicity by microscope light during surgery may be achieved by reducing the light intensity, using filters and by avoiding foveal exposure to intense light by tilting the microscope towards the surgeon.

Use of certain medications may cause photo-sensitization of the retina. These are, phenothiazine, allopurinol, haematoporphyrin, and hydroxychloroquine the surgeon should avoid using higher intensity of microscope light in the patients who are receiving these medications and also reduce exposure time to light during surgery.

# REFERENCES :

1. Irvine SR. A newly defined vitreous syndrome following cataract surgery. *Am J Ophthalmol.* 1953;36:599-619.

2. Gass JDM, Norton EWD. Cystoid macular edema and papilledema following cataract extraction: A fluorescein fundoscopic and angiographic study. *Arch Ophthalmol.* 1966;76:646-661.

3. Hitchings RA, Chrisholm IH, Bird AC. Aphakic macular edema, incidence and pathogenesis. *Invest Ophthalmol.* 1975;14:68-74.

4. Wright PL, Wilkinson CP, Balyeat HD, et al. Angiographic cystoid macular edema after posterior chamber lens implantation. *Arch Ophthalmol.* 1988;106:740-746.

5. Gass JDM. *Stereoscopic Atlas of Macular Diseases*, 4th ed. St Louis, Mo; 1997.

6. Flach AJ, Stegman RC, Graham J, et al. Prophylaxis of aphakic cystoid macular edema without corticosteroids. *Ophthalmology.* 1990;97:1253-1258.

7. Taylor Dm, Sachs SW, Stern AL. Aphakic cystoid macular edema: Long term clinical observations. *Surv Ophthalmol.* 1984;28(suppl):437-41.

8. Komatsu M, Kanagami S, Shimizu K. Ultraviolet-absorbing intraocular lens vs. non-UV absorbing intraocular lens: comparison of angiographic cystoid macular edema. *J Cataract Refract Surg.* 1989;15:658-660.

9. Guyer DR, Green WR, deBustros S, Fine SL. Histopathologic features of idiopathic macular holes and cysts. *Ophthalmology.* 1990;97:1045-1051.

10. Flach AJ, Dolan, BJ, Irvine, AR. Effectiveness of ketorolac tromethamine 0.5% ophthalmic solution for chronic aphakic and pseudophakic cystoid macular edema. *Am J Ophthalmology.* 1987;103:479-486.

# Chapter 20
# PHACO SURGERY IN CHALLENGING SITUATIONS

Phaco surgery in situations which are not usually encountered is a special area of interest for the ophthalmologist. Knowledge about these special types of cases is important because, the surgeon may then decide whether to perform surgeries on these special cases or to refer them to more experienced surgeons at a super speciality center to tackle them. It is worth knowing how to perform surgeries in these special situations. Some of the situations do not require extra equipments or facilities; others require specific instruments and techniques. Whenever, the appropriate facilities or tools to perform surgeries on these special and challenging cases are not available, early referral is recommended for appropriate management.

**The special Challenging situations are:**

A.  Small pupil cases
B.  Cataract with iritis
C.  Floppy iris syndrome
D.  Posterior polar cataract
E.  Psudoexfoliation syndrome and Weak Zonular cases
F.  Phaco surgery in Myopia
G.  Cataract surgery in glaucoma patients
H.  Pediatric cataract surgery

All these conditions must be diagnosed in the preoperative visit and diagnosis confirmed before planning for the surgery. Meticulous pre operative examination with history taking is important to diagnose and plan surgery in all these special cases. If individual situation is encountered during surgery, the case should be managed in the best and appropriate manner. The descriptions regarding the management of the challenging situations are not complete and the surgeon may decide to manage the situation as required according to individual personal experience.

# Chapter 20 A

# SMALL PUPIL CASES

A well dilated pupil increases the ease of cataract surgery; it is difficult to perform cataract surgery on any patient with pupil size less than 5 mm

During the pre-operative assessment, dilatation of the pupil is a very important parameter to be observed, as well as diagnosis of the cause of a poorly dilating pupil.

If the pupil does not dilate fully, performing phaco surgery is going to be difficult. It is also important to remember not to dilate the pupil 48 hours before the surgery and with strong dilating agents like atropine, homatropine or Cyclopentolate. In that case, the pupil will not dilate fully on subsequent attempt on the surgical day.

**The causes for small miotic pupil are:**

1. Senile iris atrophy
2. Diabetes Mellitus
3. Traumatic iris atrophy
4. Uveitis or Iritis with posterior Synechiae
5. Using Miotics for Glaucoma
6. Pseudoexfoliation Syndrome
7. Congenital
8. Floppy Iris Syndrome

**If history suggests that, any of these conditions is present, pre operative small pupil is to be expected and the surgeon should be ready to combat the situation.**

**The situations where small pupil is encountered may come in two forms:**

A. Pupils which dilate preoperatively and surgery is started with a fully dilated pupil but the pupil comes down subsequently during the progress of the surgery.
B. Pre operative small pupil which fails to dilate preoperatively and also during the surgery.

There is no straight forward process to obtain a dilated pupil in every case. There are many ways this can be approached, the choice of which depends upon the surgeon and the surgical situation.

1. **Pharmacological agents**
2. **Viscoelastics**
3. **Mechanical and surgical dilation of the pupil.**

In any case, the pupil diameter must be more than 5.5 mm to perform a successful Phaco or SICS surgery.

**Pharmacological agents :** Pre operatively, the pupil is dilated with Tropicamide 1%, Phnylephrine 2.5 % and NSAID drops and this will keep the pupil dilated throughout surgery. Addition of stronger mydriatic like Cyclopentolate 1% is reserved for difficult cases.

**A. If the pupil constricts during surgery,** which happens commonly in Diabetic patients and with senile iris atrophy, consider the following options:

1. **Viscoelastic**: Injecting a good quality viscoelastic agent in the anterior chamber may be used to dilate the pupil. The problem is the pupil remains dilated as long as the viscoelastic is in the A/C and constricts as soon as it is aspirated away. In this situation, slow down the procedure and keeps on repeatedly injecting viscoelastics throughout surgery and increase the bottle height.

2. **Diluted Cardiac Adrenaline:** Half cc cardiac adrenaline diluted with half cc BSS is directly irrigated into the anterior chamber using a blunt cannula and half cc of the diluted cardiac adrenaline is injected into the irrigating BSS bottle. This dilates the pupil immediately and the surgery can be finished with no further problems. If the pupil comes down again, this can be repeated. **The anesthetist must monitor the pulse rate and cardiac status of the patient throughout the surgery.**

**The beginning surgeon may try the following steps when confronted with a small pupil during the surgical case as per Dr. Matti Vazeen's experience:**

1) Increase the bottle height at all stages of the surgery.
2) Length of the corneal tunnel is to be increased from 3 mm to 3.5 mm if small pupil is expected.
3) Use plenty of Viscoelastics specially Viscoat and make a good Capsulorhexis

4) A good hydrodissection and rotation of the nucleus is required.

5) Do not proceed to phacoemulsification until the rotation of the nucleus is ensured.

6) Perform phacoemulsification in the center of the pupil and if iris pops into the phaco tip, release this with the second instrument and stop aspiration and ultrasound immediately. Use pharmacologic agents and good quality viscoelastic like viscoat to dilate the pupil and start phaco again.

Slow motion surgery with extreme care with good quality viscoelastics will bring out good surgical result. All instruments inserted in the anterior chamber including the phaco tip, I/A tip and chopper must be visible at all times. Avoid touching the iris at all times during the surgery.

### B. Pre operative small pupil:

If the pupil fails to dilate properly during pre-operative assessment, one or the other mechanical pupil dilating methods may be necessary. It is up to the surgeon which procedure will be undertaken, but extensive practice to use the particular device is very important before using them during surgery in real life situation.

### A. Stretching the Pupil :

The pupil is stretched by using two Iris retractors one through the side port and one through the main incision. The anterior chamber must be well filled with viscoelastics. First the pupil is stretched horizontally. Next with a push pull instruments, the iris is stretched vertically. The stretch force should be strong enough to enlarge the pupil. Irrigation of the anterior chamber with diluted adrenaline after stretching will dilate the pupil enough to perform the surgery.

### B. Iris Retractors (Iris Hooks) :

These are available commercially in two forms: Disposable or metallic multi use hooks. Four hooks needs to be introduced through four stab wounds made by the 15 degree knife or Diamond knife in the four quadrants. The Iris Hooks are introduced and the stopper is placed after retracting the iris. This has to be done in the proper way, because, unless properly placed, the iris diaphragm rises up and may be damaged during phacoemulsification. While engaging the iris, the hooks are perpendicular, after the iris is engaged; the hooks are rotated parallel to the iris before stopper is tightened. Too much stretching is to be avoided; usually a 5.5 to 6 mm stretching is enough to perform phaco surgery. The iris is fed to the retractor with iris repositor.

Once the stopper block is tightened, the hook will not rotate. One retractor is placed in each quadrant and this will result in a rectangular pupil. Trypan Blue dye is used after placing the hooks and securing them so that the iris is held in dilated position.

At the end of the surgery, each hook is removed with extreme care not to damage the Iris, otherwise injury to the iris and hemorrhage may result which will spoil the surgery. Extensive practice to place the hooks properly is necessary before actually using them on patients.

### C. Pupil Ring Expanders:

These are commercially available PMMA device which enlarge the pupil without damage to the sphincter. They are difficult to introduce and remove but once in place, they can hold the Iris in dilated position. There is a new Perfect Pupil Device developed by DR. John Milverton MD which are flexible and made of flexible material Polyurethane. This device is said to be easy to introduce and remove. Another new device is developed by Dr. Boris Malyugin MD which is also easy to introduce and removed. Several other new devices have been invented which act on the same principle of expanding the iris. The surgeon needs to practice each device on cadaver eyes or other practice eyes before using them. Please refer to the product information and publications by these authors.

### D. Mini Sphincterotomies :

Small Sphincterotomies can be performed using vannas scissors introduced through the main incision. Angled micro vannas scissors are easier to use. Each cut should be very small, not more than 0.75 mm in length. First the scissors is introduced through the main incision and a cut is made at 6 O' clock position, next the scissors is rotated to make a cut at 3 O clock and 9 O'clok positions. Subincisional position is difficult to reach and this can be reached through the side port and either angled vannas scissors of micro Vitrectomy scissors should be used. Once the cuts are made, irrigation of the anterior chamber with diluted Cardiac Adrenaline will dilate the pupil adequately for phaco surgery. However, if this fails to dilate the pupil, Iris Hook is to be used. Further cuts may cause Iris bleeding and hyphaema.

### E. Sector Iridectomy :

This used to be performed a lot during the period of Intracapsular Extraction of Lens with Cryo machine. In desperate situation, a sector Iridectomy may be performed. The iris is held with Iris scissors and cut with one snip with angled vannas scissors.

Previously, De Wekers scissors used to be available for sector or peripheral Iridectomy. However, this is not a good option because, the iris ends starts to pop into the phaco tip and the rhexis has to be perfect in this situation. The surgeon has to perform very slow, careful surgery with low flow and low vacuum and every time the phaco tip is introduced, plenty of viscoelastics is to be used to keep the iris ends away from the phaco tip. Postoperatively, the iridectomy will not interfere with vision because the Iris gap is hidden behind the upper lid.

None of these procedures is easy to perform and use of these pupil dilating devices are not in common practice. Therefore, it is advisable to practice using these devices several times on Cadaver Eyes or at least goat's eyes or pig's eyes before one can perform surgery using these devices.

## REFERENCES:

1. Masket S. Relationship between postoperative pupil size and disability glare. J Cataract Refract Surg. 1992;(18):506-7.

2. Fine IH. Phacoemulsification in the presence of a small pupil. In Steinert RF (Ed.). Cataract Surgery: Technique, Complications, & Management. Philadelphia: PA, WB Saunders; 1995. pp. 199-208.

3. Masket S. Cataract surgery complicated by the miotic pupil. In: Buratto L, Osher RH, Masket S (Eds). Cataract Surgery in Complicated Cases. Thorofare, NJ: Slack; 2000. pp. 131-7.

4. Thaller VT, Kulshrestha MK, Bell K. The effect of preoperative topical flurbiprofen or diclofenac on pupil dilatation. Eye. 2000;14(Pt4):642-5.

5. Gupta VP, Dhaliwal U, Prasad N. Ketorolac tromethamine in the maintenance of intraoperative mydriasis. Ophthalmic Surg Lasers. 1997;28(9):731-8.

6. Solomon KD, Turkalj JW, Whiteside SB, et al.Topical 0.5% ketorolac vs 0.03% flurbiprofen for inhibition of miosis during cataract surgery. Arch Ophthalmol. 1997;! 15(9): 1119-22.

7. Gimbel H, Van Westenbrugge J, Cheetham JK, et al. Intraocular availability and pupillary effect of flurbiprofen and indomethacin during cataract surgery. J Cataract Refract Surg. 1996;22(4):474-9.

8. Brown RM, Roberts CW. Preoperative and postoperative use of nonsteroidal antiinflammatory drugs in cataract surgery. Insight. 1996;21(l):13-6.

9. Kershner RM. Management of the small pupil for clear corneal cataract surgery. J Cataract Refract Surg. 2002;28(10): 1826-31.

10. Shephard DM. The pupil stretch technique for miotic pupils in cataract surgery. Ophthalmic Surg. 1994;24:851-2.

11. De Juan Jr E, Hickingbotham D. Flexible iris retractors. Am J Ophthalmol. 1991;lll:766-77.

12. Nichamin LD. Enlarging the pupil for cataract extraction using flexible nylon iris retractors. J Cataract Refract Surg. 1993;19:793-6.

13. Masket S. Avoiding complications associated with iris retractor use in small pupil cataract extraction. J Cataract Refract Surg. 1996;22:168-71.

14. Benjamin Boyd. Phacoemulsification in small pupils. In The Art and Science of Cataract Surgery; Highlights of Ophthalmology. 2001.

15. Small Pupil Phacoemulsification Amar Agarwal, Soosan Jacob, Phacoemulsification, Japee – Highlights INC : 278 -383

# Chapter 20B
# CATARACT WITH IRITIS

Cataract is a major cause of reduced visual acuity in uveitis. Cataract develops as a complication of iritis for two reasons.

1) **Firstly**, cataract may develop as a direct consequence of the disease and the more severe the disease is, more quickly lens opacities develop. In the case of mild uveitis and less frequent inflammation, cataract develops slowly.

2) **Secondly**, medications used most frequently to treat uveitis like corticosteroids, immunosuppressant themselves promote lens opacification. Therefore, premature cataract develops in most uveitis patients despite good inflammatory control. The most common form of cataract which presents as a complication of Corticosteroids is Posterior subcapsular or posterior polar opacities.

Modern cataract surgery can be safely employed to treat cataract in uveitis but, the technique is more challenging, and requires careful planning before, during, and after surgery.

Some form of iritis respond to Cataract surgery better than others. Patients with Fuchs' heterochromic Cyclitis, pars planitis, and Behcet's syndrome, usually respond well to cataract surgery. The post operative inflammation is not protracted and is comparable to standard cataract surgery. Other disorders, in contrast, such as juvenile idiopathic arthritis (juvenile chronic arthritis), severe HLA-B27-associated uveitis, and granulomatous uveitis such as sarcoidosis and Vogt-Koyanagi-Harada disease, tend to produce to more severe post operative inflammation leading to posterior synechiae formation and require intensive treatment. In some case, it may be better not to implant an IOL although the Hydrophobic Acrylic IOL is reported to be safe in most of these conditions.

**Control of inflammation** due to iritis prior to cataract surgery is most important in the management of uveitis induced cataract. It is important to know how difficult it has been to control the primary uveitis inflammation. Patients with more recurrences, or those who tend to have episodes of uveitis that are more severe, will probably have greater difficulty with surgery and it will more difficult to control the post operative inflammation. The longer intraocular inflammation is controlled prior to surgery, the better. It is now accepted that, 3 months as the minimum amount of time that a patient should be without inflammation prior to cataract surgery except in phacolytic cataract with glaucoma. In Hypermature cataract, **lens induced uveitis** is one condition where control of intraocular inflammation is not essential before cataract surgery.

Every attempt should be made to understand the cause of the uveitis if possible. The visual potential of the eye is to be assessed by retina examination, Potential Acuity Meter (PAM) and optic nerve functions tests. B scan ultrasound should be obtained prior to surgery. If the systemic cause of uveitis is found out, the underlying systemic disease is to be treated.

**Preoperative considerations**:

Once the intraocular inflammation has been controlled for 3 to 6 months with corticosteroids or other immunosuppressive agents, most patients with uveitis may undergo cataract surgery. The patient and the relatives should be informed about the risk, benefits and visual prognosis after cataract surgery in these cases. This is to be noted that, 1) The surgical procedure may take slightly longer time 2) Regional local anesthesia is preferred because of longer duration of surgery whether posterior synechiae is present or not. This means that the patient will need to go home with a patch and a shield. 3) Medications will be required both before and after surgery in order to minimize the risk of postoperative inflammation and complications. The post operative recovery period may be prolonged. The visual outcome may not be as good as other patients.

**After the surgery day is finalized, 7 days before surgery the following medications are started**:

1) Topical prednisolone acetate, 1%, every 3 hours while awake, 2) oral corticosteroids, usually prednisone 0.5 mg to 1.0 mg/kg/day. 3) In addition to the oral steroids, intravenous methylprednisolone, 250 to 1000 mg, may be given. 4) NSAID eye drops is also started at the same time 5) Anti glaucoma medications should be considered in the preoperative period should there be any suspicion of Corticosteroid responders or if IOP is increased before surgery.

**Surgical Considerations**:

1. **Anesthesia** : The surgery should be started with Regional and parabulbar injection anesthesia, usual drapes and other preoperative measures are followed as the routine cases.
2. **Posterior Synechiae**: The iritis patients often have posterior synechiae and also anterior synechiae. The posterior synechiae needs to be released during surgery. After entry incision is made, this can be done in the following ways:

233

a) Inject viscoelastic under the iris until the iris is bellowed anteriorly and the synechiae is released.

b) A cannula filled with BSS or viscoelastic is used to separate the synechiae

c) The eye is filled with viscoelastic, the synechiae are separated using a spatula carefully without injury to the anterior capsule

d) An angled vannas scissors may be used to cut the synechiae if this is difficult to break.

3) **Pupil dilatation**: Preoperative mydriatic drops are of limited use to dilate the pupil if synechiae is present. However, if there is no synechiae, pupil is dilated using the preoperative mydriatic drops and cycloplegic if necessary. If synechiae are present, these are separated and intra cameral preservative free cardiac adrenalin (Epinephrine) may be used to dilate the pupil.

4) **Mechanical pupil dilating devices**: Iris stretching, Iris Hook or pupil expanding devices may be necessary to dilate the pupil in cases where adequate dilatation is not possible with pharmacological agents alone. Care is to be taken to handle the iris while using these devices because; iris in these patients is fragile and may tear very easily.

5) **The Intraocular IOL** to be implanted must be of good quality and many has been claimed to be safe and biocompatible. Heparin Coated PMMA IOL has been used with success; Hydrophobic and some Hydrophilic lenses have long track record of bio compatibility and less inflammation. All efforts must be made to place the lens in the bag.

6) **Capsulorhexis:** Usually done with Trypan Blue Dye staining of the anterior capsule.

7) **Phacoemulsification:** Good hydrodissection and one of the chopping methods is employed for nucleus removal. Many of these cataracts are soft and must be handled with care.

8) **Implantation of IOL** : Implantation of the Intraocular Lens in the bag is most important in these cases. Sulcus placement of the lens has to be avoided by all means.

9) **Periocular injection** of Steroid like Dexamethasone and triamcinolone acetonide at the end of surgery is recommended.

**Post Operative considerations:**

Following cataract surgery in patients with uveitis, the topical and oral corticosteroids that were started prior to surgery should be tapered very slowly. This usually takes 6 weeks but may be longer in patients with severe or frequently recurrent uveitis. Some patients may require additional immunosuppressive agents, such as methotrexate, azathioprine, or cyclosporine, to control the postoperative inflammation. Intraocular pressure must be measured and anti glaucoma medication added if IOP is high.

**Cystoid macula edema (CME)** CME is a common complication in patients who have an inflammatory reaction following surgery. Treatment of the CME requires topical corticosteroid or nonsteroidal anti-inflammatory drops, a periocular corticosteroid injection of triamcinolone acetonide, 40 mg. is given. In some patients, CME is refractory and results in permanent visual impairment. But early detection by OCT and treatment may limit the macular damage.

## REFERENCES

1. Okhravi N, Towler HM, Lightman SL. Cataract surgery in patients with uveitis. *Eye.* 2000;14 Pt 5:689-690

2. Muccioli C, Belfort R Jr. Cataract surgery in patients with uveitis. *Int Ophthalmol Clin.* 2000;40(2):163-173.

3. Okhravi N, Lightman SL, Towler HM. Assessment of visual outcome after cataract surgery in patients with uveitis. *Ophthalmology.* 1999;106(4):710-722

4. Rao SK, Law RW, Yu CB, et al. IOL use in children with uveitis-related cataract. *J Pediatr Ophthalmol Strabismus.* 2001;38(3):129,176

5. Lundvall A, Zetterstrom C. Cataract extraction and intraocular lens implantation in children with uveitis. *Br J Ophthalmol.* 2000;84(7):791-793

6. Krishna R, Meisler DM, Lowder CY, Estafanous M, Foster RE. Long-term follow-up of extracapsular cataract extraction and posterior chamber intraocular lens implantation in patients with uveitis. *Ophthalmology.* 1998;105(9):1765-1769.

7. Dana MR, Chatzistefanou K, Schaumberg DA, Foster CS. Posterior capsule opacification after cataract surgery in patients with uveitis. *Ophthalmology.* 1997;104(9):1387-1393

8. Jones NP. Cataract surgery in Fuchs' heterochromic uveitis: past, present, and future. *J Cataract Refract Surg.* 1996;22(2):261-268.

9. Tabbara KF, Chavis PS. Cataract extraction in patients with chronic posterior uveitis. *Int Ophthalmol Clin.* 1995;35(2):121-131.

10. Dana MR, Chatzistefanou K, Schaumberg DA, Foster CS. Posterior capsule opacification after cataract surgery in patients with uveitis. *Ophthalmology.* 1997;104(9):1387-1393.

# Chapter 20 C
# FLOPPY IRIS SYNDROME

One disturbing situation during cataract surgery is encountered while the iris flies about and prolapses through the wound or side port and tries to come into the phaco tip. This is termed Intraoperative floppy Iris Syndrome (IFIS). This is encountered in patients taking Flomax (tamsulosin hydrochloride) and other Alpha 1 antagonist preoperatively. Flomax is prescribed in patients with benign prostatic hyperplasia to relax the smooth muscle in the bladder and prostrate to permit complete emptying of the bladder. Flomax (Tamsulosin hydrochloride) acts on alpha 1A receptor sites which are present in Prostate and dilator muscles and in the Iris.

The syndrome is presented with a triad of: 1) Iris floppiness, 2) prolapse of the iris through the wound 3) poor dilatation of the iris. However, the severity of presentation is different in different individuals and may range from mild to severe forms.

Management of the condition dependents on severity of the condition, but the surgeon must be vigilant during surgery and combat the situation with multiple strategies in mind.

**The strategies employed to manage Floppy Iris syndrome are:**

1. Pharmacological dilatation
2. Viscoelastic dilatation
3. Pupil expansion rings and devices
4. Bimanual Phaco technique.
5. Conversion to ECCE or SICS

The strategies are used alone or in combination depending on the severity of the syndrome in a graded manner.

A history of using Flomax in the preoperative period should alert the surgeon about the possibility of a floppy Iris syndrome and preventive measures taken for optimum outcome.

Firstly, the patient should be advised to stop Flomax five days before surgery, although it is documented that stopping Flomax do not reduce the IFIS but this is more to remind the surgeon about the case at the surgery day and understand what to expect.

Preoperative dilation of the patient with strong Pharmacological agents like Homatropine 2 % or, Cyclopentolate 1%, Tropicamide 1% and Phynylephrine 2.5% with usual NSAID drops will allow to start the surgery with a widely dilated pupil. Entry incision should be carefully made longer, to have a good corneal valve, injection of intracameral lidocane, good quality viscoelastic for anterior Capsulorhexis is recommended.

Hydrodissection and hydrodelineation should be performed with BSS flowing directly inside the lens, not irrigating into the anterior chamber or the iris. Once nucleus rotation is achieved, low flow phaco is started with the bottle height lowered and groove is performed. At this stage, floppiness of the iris starts to show and may come and prolapse through the wound, but in moderate cases, making the groove is possible in spite of the bellowing of the iris. Once the groove is made, the phaco needle is removed from the eye. Now the pupil will constrict and prolapsed iris is reposited back using Iris repositor. Diluted Cardiac Adrenaline (Non preserved Epinephrine) injection is irrigated into the anterior chamber which will cause re dilatation of the iris. Use Healon 5 or Viscoat to keep the iris dilated. During cracking, care is to be taken not to disturb the iris with the instruments. Slow chopping with low flow and vacuum is usually successful to perform phaco in moderate density cataracts. By the time the nucleus is emulsified, the pupil usually constricts and again intracameral adrenaline infusion will dilate the pupil for Irrigation and Aspiration of the cortex.

Lens Implant thereafter is not a problem, in the presence of a pupil size 5 mm or slightly less. It is possible to implant a foldable IOL in the bag with viscoelastic used to deepen the anterior chamber.

It is important in floppy iris that the cartridge of the injection system for IOL implantation be turned bevel-up as it is introduced into the incision in order to prevent prolapse of iris into the cartridge, so that as it exits the eye and this does not allow the iris to prolapse into the mouth of the cartridge.

However, in more difficult cases, where pupil does not dilate with epinephrine, some sort of pupil dilating device is to be used. Iris hook or, use of Malyugin Ring is ideal in the cases with small pupil and the surgery is managed as a small pupil case with care to insert these devices in the anterior chamber. In the presence of a Capsulorhexis, the edge of the ring or the hook may engage the Capsulorhexis edge and cause damage the rhexis. It is better to use Trypan Blue Dye to stain the capsule before inserting the iris expanding devices so that, the device holds only the iris and not the capsule.

In floppy iris syndrome, the physical problem is a flaccid iris that will not keep the structures at a certain plane. The zonules are weak making Capsulorhexis and hydrodissection difficult. Careful slow surgery with adjusted bottle height will deliver the expected result.

**The following steps may render the surgery safe according to the experience of Dr. Mehdi Vazeen:**

These steps will allow you to proceed to the next step without complications

1) Make your corneal tunnel longer to 3.5 to 4 mm
2) Use extra Viscoelastic of good quality like Viscoat during Capsulorhexis and look for weak zonules and adjust your surgery accordingly.
3) Take a long time in hydrodissection and ensure that the nucleus rotates freely before starting the phaco.
4) Push back the iris with viscoelastic while phaco probe is inserted.
5) Perform phacoemulsification with higher phaco power to reduce stress on the zonules and the phaco tip must be within clear visibility at all times. You are actually trying to reduce stress on the zonules.
6) If the iris prolapse and move toward the phaco tip, stop aspiration and phacoemulsification immediately and use more viscoelastic to start again. The key point is to be slow and deliberate in your movements.

If you follow the steps, you should be able to perform safe surgery in most of these small pupils, floppy iris cases with weak zonules and get good results.

## BIMANUAL PHACO

For more expert surgeons, who are competent in bimanual technique of phaco surgery, this technique is advocated, since in bimanual technique the incisions are smaller and the iris does not get the opportunity to prolapse into the wound. With the use of Iris Hook or the Malyugin ring or Morcher Pupil Expander Ring the pupil is held in dilated position and a bi manual technique gives a very safe phaco surgery, but requires an expert surgeon proficient in these techniques.

Early recognition of the syndrome and interfering adequately and timely gives the optimum surgical result in these difficult cases. They reduce the challenges and the complications associated with performing cataract surgery on patients having Flomax.

## REFERENCES :

1. Vasavada AR, Raj SM. Inside-out delineation. J Cataract Refract Surg. 2004;30(6):1167-1169.
2. Chang DF, Campbell JR. Intraoperative floppy iris syndrome associated with tamsulosin (Flomax). J Cataract Refract Surg.2005;31:664-73
3. Bell CM, Hatch WV, Fischer HD, et al. Association between tamsulosin and serious ophthalmic adverse events in older men following cataract surgery. JAMA. 2009;301:1991-6.
4. Fine IH, Hoffman RS. Phacoemulsification in the presence of pseudoexfoliation: Challenges and options. J Cataract Refract Surg. 1997;23(2):160-165.
5. Chang DF, Osher RH, Wang L, et al. Prospective multicenter evaluation of cataract surgery in patients taking tamsulosin (Flomax). Ophthalmology. 2007;! 14:957-64.
6. Masket S, Belani S. Combined preoperative topical atropine sulfate 1% and intracameral nonpreserved epinephrine hydrochloride 1:4000 [corrected] for management of intraoperative floppy-iris syndrome. J Cataract Refract Surg. 2007;33:580-2.

# Chapter 20 D
# POSTERIOR POLAR AND POSTERIOR SUBCAPSULAR CATARACT

Posterior Polar cataract is a clinical entity where a disc like Opacity is present at the center of the lens. This may be located at the Posterior pole either at the posterior sub capsular region or directly on the posterior capsule. The cortical fibers may be actually adherent to the opacity on the posterior capsule or the opacity may be located on the posterior pole just in front of the posterior capsule, not adherent to it.

The Posterior subcapsular opacity may be inherited as congenital autosomal dominant entity or acquired due to toxic agents and may be steroid induced cataract. Similar type of posterior subcapsular cataract is also encountered in patients receiving Chemotherapy, Renal Dialysis, High Myopia, Retinitis Pigmentosa, Gyrate Atrophy of the Choroid and other degenerative conditions.

Primary congenital Posterior Polar Cataract presents as disc shaped opacity in the posterior cortex, either stationary opacity and the overlying cataract may be nuclear sclerosis type. Or the opacity may present as progressive opacity with spokes radiating from the central posterior subcapsular opacity. Cataract secondary to corticosteroids and related medications develop as posterior polar and subcapsular opacities with clear cortex and nucleus. Gradually as the nuclear opacities develop, vision may reduce and the patient complains of progressive glare and dispersion of light. Surgical management of all these types of cataract is the same and therefore described together.

Posterior Subcapsular cataract poses a special challenge for phacoemulsification or SICS and has to be handled in a specific manner. The surgeon must be careful and vigilant during surgery, so that surgical complications and posterior capsule rupture can be avoided.

**Anesthesia :** Parabulber local anesthesia with massage of the globe to reduce Intraocular pressure is preferred to reduce posterior vitreous pressure. Topical anesthesia may used by experienced surgeons. Preoperative light compression of the globe with super pinky for 05 minutes before starting the surgery with topical or regional anesthesia may be helpful. This is to reduce positive vitreous pressure which may pose a problem for hydro procedures in this type of cataract.

**Entry and Rhexis :** Clear corneal incision entry to the eye with standard 2.8 mm blade and a side port with a 15 degree knife is performed. The rhexis should not be more than 5 mm in diameter. Bigger rhexis is to be avoided so that, should a rent in posterior capsule be detected, the lens can be placed in the Sulcus over the anterior capsular rhexis. But too small Capsulorhexis is to be avoided because that will exert extra stress on the posterior capsule during hydro procedures.

**Hydro delineation and Hydrodissection:** This is the most important step of the surgery. Hydrodissection is to be avoided. Attempt to hydrodissection may cause a rent in the posterior capsule. The simple reason is, the opacity is directly on or just above the posterior pole and there is not enough space for the fluid wave to traverse forward and also the opaque plaque is non compliant and cannot move up even fraction of a millimeter. Therefore, any attempt to move the fluid through this space causes the fluid wave to get misdirected and ruptures the posterior capsule. However careful hydrodissection is possible by sending small pulses of fluid to break the adhesions at the posterior pole. **Hydrodelineation** can be performed in two ways:

1) **Standard hydrodelineation** using a Right Angle Cannula and going to the desired depth into the substance of the nucleus so that the fluid wave passes above the posterior polar opacity.

2) **Inside out Hydrodelineation** as described by Dr. Abhay Vasavada is a very clever way to hydro delineate at the correct plane where the surgeon wants the fluid wave to pass.

3) **Femto-Delineation :** Recently, Dr. Abhay Vasavada has described a new procedure to be able to delineate the Nucleus to the desired depth using Femtosecond Laser and OCT.

Hydrodelineation is the most important step for success in this type of cataract surgery. Direct hydrodelineation can be performed by directing the bent side of the right angle cannula in the substance of the lens where the delineation is expected and then inject fluid, a fluid wave will pass through the substance of the lens and a golden ring will be visible. Stop any further injection of fluid as soon as the golden ring is visible.

**Inside out hydrodelineation** as described by Dr. Vasavada involves making a central trench in the nucleus, viscoelastic is injected into the anterior chamber before removing the phaco tip to avoid forward movement of the posterior capsule. The hydrodissection cannula is introduced through the main incision and placed on the right side of the trench at the appropriate depth to create the delineation required protecting the posterior capsular opacity. Delineation is produced by the fluid passing inside out and visible as a golden ring. In this procedure precise epinucleus bowl necessary to cushion and to protect the posterior capsule is delineated and safe surgery can be performed. Please refer to the original article by Dr. Vasavada for details of this procedure.

**Rotation of the nucleus:** Nucleus rotation is avoided to minimize mechanical stress on the capsule.

**Phacoemulsification of the nucleus:** The nucleus phacoemulsification needs to be performed not by cracking, but by Chop in Situ and stop chop and stuff method. If the nucleus is soft, this can be removed by chip and flip technique. Care is taken not to disturb the epinuclear shell which may be a bulky shell of epinucleus and cortex. This is cleared by Irrigation and aspiration after the removal of nucleus.

**Hydro separation of the cortex:** The phaco tip is removed from the eye and what remains is the epinuclear- cortical bowl where the nucleus is removed. Next, the hydrodissection cannula is taken again and small amount of BSS is irrigated in the different quadrants under the capsule to separate the cortex and capsular adhesions in all the quadrants. The spray of fluid should be weak and not to traverse beneath the subcapsular opacity, but just to reach the equator of the lens, the subincisional area can be reached with a J shaped cannula or entering through the side port. This loosens up the whole epinuclear- cortical bowl from the anterior portion of the capsule. This is then removed by striping with the Phaco needle at low vacuum and low flow. Slow striping action will remove most of the epinucleus and attached cortex. The remainder of the cortex can be removed with I/A cannula or a Simco Cannula. Simco cannula at this stage may give more control of aspiration and flow for the beginning surgeon. If the opacity on the posterior capsule is removed and the opacity is not adherent to the posterior capsule, standard irrigation and aspiration handpiece is used to strip and clear the remainder of the cortical mater.

**At the end of cortex removal:** An Intact clear posterior capsule may remain or there may be an opacity sticking to the posterior capsule. It is dangerous to polish and remove this small posterior capsular opacity which should be left as it is.

**IOL implantation:** Foldable IOL is implanted in the bag. If there is a posterior capsular opacity that did not come with the cortex by striping, it is left behind to be removed by YAG LASER posterior capsulotomy after the eye has healed, usually 3 months after surgery.

**Posterior Capsular Dehiscence:** If a posterior capsular dehiscence is detected, gentle vitrectomy is performed to remove any vitreous from the anterior chamber and the IOL is implanted at the sulcus. In some rare cases the posterior capsule may be deficient at a very small area. It is not necessary to be worried about this very small hole in the posterior capsule and if there is no vitreous in the anterior chamber, the IOL may be implanted in the bag or the sulcus as possible. The viscoelastic is removed with low flow and aspiration taking time not to put pressure or stress on the posterior capsule.

References :

1. Posterior Polar Cataract Abhay R Vasavada, Shetal M Raj Chapter 41 Pp 331 -332 Phacoemulsification Fourth Edition Jaypee – Highlights, 2012

2. Tulloh CG. Hereditary posterior polar cataract with report of a pedigree. Br J Ophthalmol. 1955;39(6):374-9.

3. Osher RH, Yu BC, Koch DD. Posterior polar cataracts: : predisposition to intraoperative posterior capsular rupture. Journal of Cataract and Refractive Surgery. 1990;16:157-62.

4. Duke-Elder S. Posterior polar cataract. System of Ophthalmology: Normal and Abnormal Development, CongenitalDeformities. St Louis, MO: CV Mosby; 1964. pp. 723-6.

5. Vasavada AR, Singh R. Phacoemulsification with posterior polar cataract. Journal of Cataract and Refractive Surgery. 1999;25:238-45.

6. Eshagian J. Human posterior subcapsular cataracts. Trans Ophthalmol Soc UK. 1982;102:364-8.

7. Lee MW, Lee YC. Phacoemulsification of posterior polar cataracts—a surgical challenge. British Journal of Ophthalmology. 2003;87:1426-7.

8. Liu Y, Liu Y, Wu M, et al. Phacoemulsification in eyes with posterior polar cataract and foldable intraocular lens implantation. Yan Ke Xue Bao. 2003; 19(2):92-4.

9. Fine IH, Packer M, Hoffman RS. Management of posterior polar cataract. Journal of Cataract and Refractive Surgery. 2003 ;29:16-9.

10. Fine,Cortico-cleaving hydrodissection. Journal of Cataract and Refractive Surgery. 1992;18:508-12.

11. Vasavada AR, Raj SM. Inside-Out delineation. Journal of Cataract Refract Surgery. 2004;30:1167-9.

12. Allen D, Wood C. Minimizing risk to the capsule during surgery for posterior polar cataract. Journal of Cataract and Refractive Surgery. 2002; 28:742-4.

# Chapter 20 E
# PSEUDOEXFOLIATION SYNDROME_AND WEAK ZONULE CASES

Management of cataract when there is zonular weakness and zonular deficiency is a challenging task. The surgical procedure requires special skill and special judgment. With the recent advancement in instrumentations and technique it is now possible to perform Phaco surgery and implant an IOL in these difficult patients. During the period of an Intracapsular extraction of lens, weak zonules was an advantage and we would wait for a cataract to be mature enough to have a weak zonules, so that the whole lens would come out with the capsule held by the cryo probe. When the surgery changed to Extracapsular Cataract Extraction with IOL implant in 1990, we learned to make a big incision and instead of expression of nucleus, we learned to pull the nucleus out of the bag into the anterior chamber and deliver the nucleus by Viscoexprerssion so that extra stress on the zonules is reduced. Performing phaco in the weak zonules cases was difficult and was avoided until 1994 or 1996 when Capsular tension ring was described and popularized by Dr. Hara et al and Dr. Nagamoto.

Causes of weak zonules: Weakness of the zonules can be encountered in a number of situations.

1. Pseudo exfoliation cataract with or without glaucoma
2. Hypermature Cataract
3. Trauma
4. Marfan's Syndrome and similar conditions.
5. High Myopia and Buphthalmos
6. Diseases like Retinitis Pigmentosa and Uveitis

Whatever be the cause of weakness of the zonules, the most important danger is zonular dialysis and dislocation of the entire lens and prolapse of vitreous into the anterior chamber. Therefore the surgery is to be designed so that minimum or no stress falls on the zonules during the surgical maneuvers.

a) **Anesthesia**: Because of the uncertainty of complications during the surgery, long lasting anesthesia either Peribulber and regional injection anesthesia or General Anesthesia is preferred. Intracameral injection of xylocaine is avoided because there is a possibility that the anesthetic may pass to the posterior segment and cause retinal toxicity. The eye is prepared and draped as a routine case.

b) **Incision:** The main incision site is to be chosen on the opposite side of the area of zonular dehiscence. This ensures that all subsequent steps can be performed without stress on the already weak zonular area.

c) **Capsulorhexis and hydrodissection**: The Capsulorhexis is started in the area of intact zonules with the help of a good viscoelastic. It is better to avoid cystitome to create the rhexis; a Capsulorhexis forceps gives better control of the force of pull along the weaker areas. Hydrodissection should be aimed at cortical cleaving hydrodissection with breaking the capsulocortical adhesions and as complete as possible so that nucleus rotation can be achieved by gentle movements.

d) **Insertion of the Capsular Tension Ring:** Various designs of CTR Rings are available like Morcher CTR Ring(FCI Ophthalmics), ReFORM CTR (Alcon), StabilEyes CTR (AMO), (Cionni CTR (FCI Ophthalmics). The Capsule Tension Ring or simply CTR ring like the Morcher Endocapsular ring is inserted with a guide suture. After insertion, the ring secures the bag against the ciliary sulcus and thus helps to perform the surgery without stress on the zonules. The device is loaded into the injector and inserted through the rhexis and as it opens up, the device secures the capsular bag. Good quality viscoelastic should be used to gently inflate the bag before insertion of the CTR.

e) **Nucleus removal and aspiration of the cortex**: These steps are performed in slow motion and reduced flow with minimum turbulence of the anterior chamber. The aspiration and flow rate is reduced by lowering the bottle height. This is the only situation when anterior chamber phaco should be performed with the aid of a cohesive viscoelastic to protect endothelium. After the initial groove is made, the nucleus is cracked and the half nucleus is pulled to the center and brought into the anterior chamber to be emulsified. Chopping and rotation of the nucleus in the bag is avoided, all chopping and aspiration should be done outside the bag, in the anterior chamber or at the Iris plane. Aspiration of the cortical mater is done with deliberate movements with minimum vacuum and flow rate by lowering the bottle height.

f) **Implantation of IOL and viscoelastic removal:** The Foldable IOL is implanted in the bag, Optic size should be large about 7 mm and the IOL overall size should be 13.mm. After implantation of the IOL, rotation of the IOL is avoided. Just insert the IOL in the bag and keep it in the position it assumes without dialing. Removal of viscoelastic should be performed with caution without any turbulence in the anterior chamber.

The problem in pseudo exfoliation and weak zonules is that it is difficult to perform Capsulorhexis, hydrodissection and phacoemulsification in these cases. The indications that the zonules are weak are that as you do Capsulorhexis, you will see folds and wrinkles on the capsular surface as if the capsule is redundant. The surgical steps to counter these physical properties are 1) Use plenty of viscoelastics and perform rhexis with forceps by grasping and regrasping the capsule in slow turns. 2) Slow and complete hydrodissection so that nucleus rotation is achieved easily. 3) During phacoemulsification, reduced flow and gentle movement in the anterior chamber in addition to using the CTR rings. 4) The CTR ring should be secured by suturing this to the sclera.

With modern machines, CTR ring and improved mechanics, it is possible to perform safe surgery in patients with pseudoexfoilation, damaged zonules, Traumatic zonular dehiscence and Marfans Syndrome. This requires skilled and experienced surgeon and appropriate use of the instruments and equipments.

## REFERENCE :

1. Nagamoto T, Bissen-Miyajima H. A ring to support the capsular bag after continuous curvilinear capsulorhexis. Cataract Refract Surg. 1994;20:417-20.

2. Menapace R, Findl O, Georgopoulos M, et al. The capsular tension ring: Designs, applications, and techniques. J Cataract Refract Surg. 2000;898-912.

3. Strenn K, Menapace R, Vass C, Capsular bag shrinkage implantation of an open loop silicone lens and a polyr methacrylate capsule tension ring. J Cataract Refract 1997;23:1543-7.

4. Groessl SA, Anderson CJ. Capsular tension ring in a patient with Weill-Marchesani syndrome. J Cataract and Refract Surg. 1998;24:1164-5.

5. Gimbel HV, Sun R, Heston JP. Management of zonular dialysis in phacoemulsification and IOL implantation using the capsular tension ring. Ophthalmic Surg Lasers. 1997;28:273-81

6. Sun R, Gimbel HV. In vitro evaluation of the efficacy of the capsular tension ring for managing zonular dialysis in cataract surgery. Ophthalmic Surg Lasers. 1998;29:502

## Chapter 20 F
# PHACO SURGERY IN MYOPIA

Phacoemulsification in Myopic patients requires some special considerations because of the potential operative and post operative challenges they pose. Lens extraction surgery with and IOL implant can cure any amount of Myopia and Astigmatism and these patients are relieved from shortsightedness with its attendant disadvantages. The surgery is performed for:

1. Age related cataract in Myopic patients
2. Clear Lens extraction for the correction of Myopia

**Pre Operative considerations:**

In addition to the usual work up for cataract surgery, full examination of the periphery of the retina to locate any weak areas or myopic degeneration is to be elucidated. If there are any degenerative areas in the retina, this needs to be treated before phacoemulsification.

While performing biometry, it is to be noted that, Ultrasound A scan biometry may give false axial length and the post operative refraction may result in Hypermetropia. Optical device like IOL master gives a more accurate IOL power calculation. The patient should be corrected to give -0.5 D to -1.00 D postoperative myopia rather than emmetropia.

**Patients are placed on NSAID drops twice daily four days prior to surgery for the following reasons:**

(1) Prevention of small pupil during surgery
(2) Analgesia and patient comfort
(3) Reduction in the postoperative inflammatory response
(4) Prevention of postoperative cystoid macular edema (CME).

**During Surgery**

**The problem with High Myopic patients is that, there is more space in the anterior chamber and also you get less support and therefore, there is more vaulting of the nucleus while doing phaco. Therefore, you should decrease the bottle height and use less viscoelastics. The corneal tunnel should be 3.5 to 4 mm for better stability of the anterior chamber.**

In myopic patients the anterior chamber depth is large, which allows for more working space during phacoemulsification. However, the infusion pressure from the phaco handpiece can cause over-inflation of the anterior chamber and a tendency to push the entire iris-lens diaphragm posterior. Because of this very deep anterior chamber, the pupil tends to come down and the surgery becomes difficult due to the fact that, the depth of focus of the microscope cannot cope with the increased depth of the anterior chamber and visibility of the surgical field is reduced thus it becomes uncomfortable for both the surgeon and the patient. The bottle height may be lowered to reduce flow which reduces the depth of the anterior chamber.

Patients with myopia are at a higher risk for postoperative retinal detachment which is caused by unstable Anterior Chamber and surge during surgery. If the A/C collapses during surgery for any reason, this creates traction on the vitreous base causing the weak retinal periphery to break and cause retinal detachment. When the phaco probe or the I/A probe is withdrawn abruptly from the eye, the anterior chamber becomes shallow and pulls the iris lens diaphragm upwards and the vitreous base moves forward causing traction at the base of the vitreous. To prevent this, the anterior chamber is filled with viscoelastic or BSS through the side port before the Phaco probe or I/A probe is withdrawn to keep the anterior chamber pressurized to prevent collapse. The other way to prevent collapse is to activate continuous irrigation mode of the machine by moving the foot to the right on the foot paddle and remove the phaco probe out of the anterior chamber slowly. Shallowing of the anterior chamber should be minimized during surgery with all the available options to minimize surge.

These patients tend to have postoperative inflammation and use of antibiotics, steroids and NSAID drops in the postoperative period is indicated.

Because of the fact that myopic patients tend to have thinner and more elastic sclera, and sometimes corneal thickness is less than that of emmetropic patients, there may be a higher risk of incision leakage; this should be examined at the end of surgery. One stitch should be placed if there is wound leak or instability of the wound. The length of the corneal tunnel is therefore important and should be 3.5 to 4 mm to get a better stabilization of the anterior chamber and postoperative wound closure.

During the post-operative period a dilated Fundus examination is indicated in order to search for possible retinal breaks or weakness that may have been created during surgery. Repeated measurement of IOP in postoperative follow-up is important because many of the myopic patients develop glaucoma due to the use of steroid eye drops.

Cataract Surgery or Clear Lens Extraction in Myopia is a challenging task but the patients are very happy candidates for surgery because of the dramatic refractive outcome is these cases. The patient will have high anisometropia postoperatively and the second eye should be operated as soon as possible to restore emmetropia in both eyes.

## REFERENCES :

1. Brown NAHill AR Cataract: the relation between myopia and cataract morphology. *Br J Ophthalmol* 1987;71405- 414

2. Wong TYFoster PJJohnson GJSeah SK Refractive errors, axial ocular dimensions, and age-related cataracts: the Tanjong Pagar survey. *Invest Ophthalmol Vis Sci* 2003;441479- 1485

3. Hoffer KJ Axial dimension of the human cataractous lens. *Arch Ophthalmol* 1993;111914- 918

4. Wensor MMcCarty CATaylor HR Prevalence and risk factors of myopia in Victoria, Australia. *Arch Ophthalmol* 1999;117658- 663

5. Younan CMitchell PCumming RGRochtchina EWang JJ Myopia and incident cataract and cataract surgery: the Blue Mountains Eye Study. *Invest Ophthalmol Vis Sci* 2002;433625- 3632

6. Kaufman BJSugar J Discrete nuclear sclerosis in young patients with myopia. *Arch Ophthalmol* 1996;1141178- 1180

## Chapter 20 G

# CATARACT IN GLAUCOMA PATIENTS

Chronic simple Glaucoma and narrow angle glaucoma poses a management problem in cataract patients. There is no generalized rule of procedures for the management of Glaucoma in cataract patients. Different surgeons will address the problem in different ways. There are a number of procedures to choose from and each surgical procedure is a standard surgery, it is up to the surgeon to use the best suited procedure for the patient.

First approach when a patient presents with cataract and glaucoma is the assessment of pre operative status of Glaucoma, the extent of optic nerve damage due to Glaucoma, type of Glaucoma and then decide what approach will be appropriate for the individual patient.

It is now established that, Cataract surgery alone reduces intraocular pressure from 2 to 8 mm Hg in diagnosed open angle glaucoma patients. Removal of the lens may be curative in many narrow angle glaucoma patients.

Combined surgery reduces intraocular pressure more than cataract surgery alone.

1.  If the patient has IOP in the region of 22 mm Hg and little or no optic nerve damage, Phaco with IOL implant alone will reduce the IOP to a safer level and the patient will require minimum medication to control the IOP and glaucoma.
2.  If the patient has poorly controlled Glaucoma with Visual field damage, a combined procedure is usually performed. This can be performed in many ways :
    a)  LASER Trabeculoplasty followed by cataract surgery
    b)  Phacoemulsification with Trabeculectomy
    c)  Phacoemulsification with minimally invasive Glaucoma surgery
    d)  Phacoemulsification with ExPRESS Shunt (Alcon)
    e)  Phacoemulsification with suprachoroidal shunts
    f)  Trabecular micro-bypass stent: (I-Stent) : A new procedure which gives better outcome

## PHACOEMULSIFICATION ALONE

In present day technique, standard clear corneal phacoemulsification is performed through the temporal or superior approach. This reduces the IOP by 2 to 8 mm Hg. The surgery can be performed under Topical Anesthesia. In narrow angle patients a peripheral Iridectomy may be performed.

## LASER TRABECULOPLASTY:

Pre operatively or post operatively, Laser Trabeculoplasty can further reduce IOP by about 4 to 8 mm Hg. It is possible to control IOP in patients with medically controlled glaucoma by Phacoemulsification and Laser Trabeculoplasty. Use of one kind of medication for further control of IOP in the post operative period is well tolerated by the patients.

## Combined phacoemulsification and trabeculectomy

Combined phacoemulsification with Glaucoma surgery is reserved for those patients where the IOP is uncontrolled and the patients are non compliant to use medications.

## SINGLE SITE PHACOEMULSIFICATION WITH TRABECULECTOMY:

The problem of performing combined Trabeculectomy and cataract surgery is the bleb formation, increased risk of infection and post operative astigmatism. However, if the preoperative IOP control is poor and there is glaucoma damage to the optic nerve before cataract surgery, combined procedure is more effective in controlling IOP than cataract surgery alone or other procedures. The single site surgery is performed to avoid two surgeries and minimize the post operative astigmatism. A limbus based or fornix based conjunctival flap is created. Partial thickness scleral flap is designed; the width of the flap is 4 to 5 mm and dissected up to the blue area of corneo-scleral limbus. The anterior chamber is entered below the scleral flap into the cornea making the corneal valve for phaco surgery. Direct entry to anterior chamber is to be avoided because this will cause iris prolapse and makes phaco surgery difficult.

The phacoemulsification and IOL implantation is performed as a routine procedure. The sclerectomy and Iridectomy is performed after completion of the phaco surgery. However, the sclerectomy is difficult to perform than standard trabeculectomy. It is recommended to use a sharp blade or diamond knife to perform sclerectomy and a punch is very useful to remove the desired amount of scleral tissue and perform a good sclerectomy for effective drainage. The Iridectomy is performed using a micro iris forceps and angled vannas scissors.

The scleral flap and the conjunctival flaps are sutured with right apposition, care being taken not to tie the sutures too tight. Although the surgery can be performed under topical anesthesia, the most common preferred anesthesia is peribulber injection with no pressure on the eye ball and light sedation to alleviate anxiety.

## SEPARATE SITE PHACOEMULSIFICATION AND TRABECULECTOMEY SURGERY:

In this procedure, the two surgeries are performed in two separate quadrants. Phacoemulsification is done through the temporal clear corneal approach and Trabeculectomy through the superior approach for better bleb formation.

The conjunctival flap is dissected; partial thickness scleral flap is dissected up to the limbus and left over there.

Next, clear corneal phacoemulsification is performed through temporal approach. After the IOL is implanted, the surgeon moves back to the superior site and completes Trabeculectomy.

Sclerectomy and Iridectomy are performed as in standard trabeculectomy. It is also difficult to perform the sclerectomy in this situation because, after the phaco surgery, the eye ball is soft and requires very sharp blade to cut and remove the scleral tissue. Use of diamond knife and a punch is very useful. The scleral flap and the conjunctival flap are sutured as in a standard Trabeculectomy surgery.

## CATARCT SURGERY WITH MINIMALLY INVASIVE GLAUCOMA SURGERY :

a) **Trabectome and Phaco surgery :**

Trabectome is a minimally invasive glaucoma surgery for the surgical management of glaucoma. The surgery does not create an external filtering bleb or require leaving a permanent hole in the eye as in Trabeculectomy. Trabectome (NeoMedix) is performed under direct visualization of the angle with a gonioscopy lens and removes a 60-to 120-degree strip of the trabecular meshwork and the inner wall of Schlemm's canal with electrocautery. The goal is to achieve direct flow of aqueous into the canal of shelemm and then into the collector channels. The trabectome electo-surgical handpiece opens access to the eye's natural drainage system. This procedure is performed through a small incision and phaco surgery can be performed after the Trabectome surgery is performed. In expert hands, this is a safe surgery and reduces IOP by about 4 to 8 mm Hg.

b) **Viscocanalostomy and Phaco surgery**:

Viscocanalostomy is a type of non-penetrating filtration surgery and reduces intraocular pressure by dissecting a superficial scleral flap and excising a deeper partial-thickness scleral flap below the superficial flap. The aqueous humor diffuses and drains from the anterior chamber into the subconjunctival space or through Schlemm's canal into which a high-density viscoelastic substance has been injected. The superficial flap is sutured in place at the end of the procedure.

Phaco surgery is performed through a separate Clear Corneal Temporal approach before the Viscocanalostomy is performed.

The advantage of the procedure is that it does not leave a bleb and the IOP reduction is between 4 to 8mm Hg.

c) **Ex PRESS filtration shunt and Phaco surgery:**

This is a relatively new device used in combination of a trabeculectomy procedure; the ExPRESS filtration device shunts aqueous fluid from the anterior chamber into a subconjunctival bleb. The device adds to trabeculectomy a greater control of outflow. The ExPRESS device is 3 mm long, with an external diameter of about 400 microns, and it is inserted beneath a scleral flap in a procedure like Trabeculectomy without performing the scerectomy and iridectomy. The shunt is inserted under the scleral flap and this causes guarded drainage of aqueous from the anterior chamber.

The lamellar dissection of sclera is performed as in trabeculectomy. Clear Corneal temporal approach phaco surgery is performed and IOL implanted.

The Ex PRESS shunt is then inserted under the partial thickness scleral flap and the flap is sutured. The conjunctiva is also sutured at the end of the surgery.

d) **Trabecular micro-bypass stent:** This is a FDA approved medical device called I stent and is a new procedure in Glaucoma surgery. The I stent is implanted with Gonioscopic guidance and controls IOP by 4 to 8 mm Hg in glaucoma patients. In this combined procedure, phacoemulsification is performed by temporal clear corneal incision and the Stent placement is done next in the same setting.

Co existing glaucoma and cataract is difficult to manage and individual patients are to be evaluated separately. Each patient is to be managed according to the preoperative assessment of Glaucoma and target Intraocular Pressure to be achieved. None of these new glaucoma surgeries is easy to perform and requires special training and skill. It is advised that the surgeon learns the particular surgical procedure and practice them well before using any of these implants.

## PHACOLYTIC AND PHACOANAPHYLACTIC GLAUCOMA AND CATARACT:

Phacolytic and Phacoanaphylactic glaucoma happens in Hypermature and Morgagnian Cataract. Upon diagnosis it an urgent situation to reduce IOP as soon as possible and cataract surgery is performed to remove the offending lens and cortical mater.

Immediate hospitalization is necessary because the IOP rises rapidly to the region of 60 mmHg and causes damage to the Optic Nerve and if not relieved quickly, may cause optic atrophy and permanent blindness.

Immediate infusion of Mannitol at least 500 ml to rapidly reduce the Intraocular Pressure and preparation of surgery as soon as possible will save the eye and vision. SICS or ECCE with PC IOL implant under Mannitol cover may be performed. Performing phaco on these hard cataracts, sometimes with liquefied cortical mater is very difficult. Small Incision Cataract Surgery (SICS) with a peripheral Iridectomy reduces the intraocular pressure and controls Glaucoma very well. The Intraocular pressure is usually controlled post operatively but, due to the possibility of rise of IOP and inflammation in the immediate post operative period, the patient is put on oral Acetazolamide and potent topical steroids during the post operative period.

Glaucoma with cataract is a special situation and whether the patient presents with open angle glaucoma with cataract or, angle closure glaucoma with cataract they need to be evaluated meticulously both for glaucoma and cataract. The management of each condition is different and separate but not independent of each other. The surgeon should evaluate the situation and act appropriately.

## References :

1. Gedde SJ. Results from the tube versus trabeculectomy study. Middle East Afr J Ophthalmol. 2009 Jul;16(3):107-11.
2. Kleinmann G, Katz H, Pollack A, Schechtman E, Rachmiel R, Zalish M. Comparison of trabeculectomy with mitomycin C with or without phacoemulsification and lens implantation. Ophthalmic Surg Lasers. 2002;33(2):102-108.

3. Poley BJ, Lindstrom RL, Samuelson TW, Schulze R Jr. Intraocular pressure reduction after phacoemulsification with intraocular lens implantation in glaucomatous and nonglaucomatous eyes: evaluation of a causal relationship between the natural lens and open-angle glaucoma. J Cataract Refract Surg. 2009;35(11):1946-1955.

4. Francis BA, Minckler D, Dustin L, et al; Trabectome Study Group. Combined cataract extraction and trabeculotomy by the internal approach for coexisting cataract and open-angle glaucoma: initial results. J Cataract Refract Surg. 2008;34(7):1096-1103.

5. Maris PJ, Ishida K, Netland PA. Comparison of trabeculectomy with Ex-PRESS miniature glaucoma device implanted under sclera flap. J Glaucoma. 2007 Jan;16(1):14-9

6. Lai JS, Tham CC, Chan JC. The clinical outcomes of cataract extraction by phacoemulsification in eyes with primary angle-closure glaucoma (PACG) and co-existing cataract: a prospective case series. J Glaucoma. 2006;15(1):47-52

7. Shingleton B, Tetz M, Korber N. Circumferential viscodilation and tensioning of Schlemm canal (canaloplasty) with temporal clear corneal phacoemulsification cataract surgery for open-angle glaucoma and visually significant cataract: one-year results. J Cataract Refract Surg. 2008;34(3):433-440.

8. Hayashi K, Hayashi H, Nakao F, Hayashi F. Changes in anterior chamber angle width and deep  after intraocular lens implantation in eyes with glaucoma. Ophthalmology. 2000;107(4):69

9. Craven ER, KatzU Wells JM, Giamporcaro JE, I Stent Study Group ; ; Cataract surgery with trabecular micro-bypass stent implantation in patients with mild-to-moderate open-angle  glaucoma and cataract: two-year follow-up,. J Cataract Refract Surg. 2012 Aug;38(8):1339-45.

## Chapter 20 H
# PEADIATRIC CATARACT SURGERY

Management of pediatric cataract is a challenge for the ophthalmologist, the parents and the all the caregivers. Congenital cataract may be present at birth, or may present as developmental lens opacities later in childhood. Amblyopia and nystagmus are the two dangers in pediatric cataract.

Surgery of childhood cataract depends upon the cause and type of cataract, age of onset and age of presentation, level of preexisting amblyopia, type of refractive correction affordable by the parents, and surgical facilities available.

This requires special skill on the part of the surgeon, understanding of the parents and cooperation of the supporting staff, anesthesiologist and primary care pediatrician.

## INCIDENCE :

Cataract is one of the major causes of preventable blindness. The incidence of cataract during infancy has been estimated to be 3 to 6 per 10,000 births. Approximately 45% of these cataracts are unilateral; 55 % are bilateral. The total incidence of cataract in childhood is more than this figure. Other causes of childhood blindness are trauma, corneal opacity due to measles and vitamin A deficiency, metabolic disorders, radiation treatment, and corticosteroid induced cataract.

## HERIDITY :

Congenital cataract is most commonly inherited as Autosomal dominant, but may also be autosomal recessive and X linked. Many cases are sporadic and may present as unilateral cataract.

## INTRAUTERINE INFECTION:

Congenital Rubella infection in the first trimester of pregnancy may cause cataract and is present in about 15 % of cases.

Other infections that can cause congenital cataract are, CMV, Toxoplasma, HSV and vericella during pregnancy.

## CHROSOMAL ABNORMALITIES:

Down's syndrome is associated with cataract and often with amblyopia. Other abnormalities like Trisomy 13 and 18 are also associated with cataracts.

**SYSTEMIC CONDITIONS**, like Galactosemia, Lowe's Syndrome and Hypoparathyroidism may be associated with cataract.

## MORPHOLOGICAL TYPES:

The morphological type of the cataract is important because, we can understand the etiology and plan for the appropriate management.

1. Lamellar: The opacity may be deep lamellar to cover the whole lens or may affect one lamella anteriorly and posteriorly.
2. Nuclear: usually inherited, the cataract affects the fetal nucleus and may be dense causing profound loss of vision.
3. Coronary : Cortical cataract that surrounds the nucleus, this is usually sporadic
4. Blue dot cataract : are usually harmless
5. Sutural : the opacity is in the anterior and posterior Y sutures, may or may not affect vision
6. Anterior polar and posterior polar cataracts are due to developmental anomalies.
7. Membranous cataracts occur when lens material is partially absorbed leaving behind a membranous opacity.

### Surgical procedures :

Many surgical procedures are adopted for treating Congenital Cataract.

a) Needling and aspiration: During 70's the eye used to be entered with a fine knife, anterior capsule punctured by the same knife. Since the cataract is soft and milky, this used to be washed out with saline or BSS through a cannula fitted on a syringe. At that time simco cannula was not available.

b) ECCE: During 80's when ECCE was practiced for adult patients, can opener anterior capsulotomy with irrigation and aspiration of the lens using a two way simco cannula was performed for the pediatric cataracts through a small incision.

c) IOL Implantation: during mid 80's to mid 90's IOL implantation was tried after ECCE and enlarging the incision to implant an IOL.

**All these procedures used to be complicated with severe post operative inflammation and development of posterior capsular opacity. The posterior capsules were cut by a knife or needle as a secondary procedure. The child's vision remained poor.**

d) The situation improved in late 90's after the availability of Heparin Coated Intraocular Lens. This reduced the inflammation and better acceptance of IOL in pediatric cases.

e) With the development of mechanized lensectomy in the mid-1980s, the mechanized lensectomy and vitrectomy for young children undergoing cataract surgery was routine in Europe and slowly came to the developing world as well.

f) With the development of Phaco machine and when it became available worldwide in 1990's, pediatric cataracts were also removed by irrigation and aspiration with the phaco machine. But implantation of an IOL was still controversial.

g) With the development of phaco machine and Hydrophobic IOL in mid 1990, IOL implantation for children gained popularity.

These procedures have all been performed for the treatment of congenital cataract. This depends upon the availability of the facilities, equipments and surgical skill at a particular country and particular situation for the management of childhood cataract.

## PRESENT DAY MANAGEMENT OF CONGENITAL CATARACT:

Management depends upon the age of presentation and type of opacity. Early surgery is advocated if congenital cataract is present at birth. Timing of surgery is crucial for the development of useful vision during the post operative period.

a) In bilateral dense cataracts, early surgery, Lensectomy with anterior vitrectomy often by the age of 6 months to prevent the development of stimulus deprivation amblyopia. Permanent sensory nystagmus develops if the surgery is delayed beyond 4 months, but considering general anesthesia is to be given, 4 to 6 months of age is a viable option.

b) Unilateral cataract requires urgent surgery often before 6 weeks of age followed by intensive anti-amblyopia therapy with occlusion and close follow up. If unilateral cataract is detected after 6 month of age, immediate surgery is performed and amblyopia treatment is pursued in spite of the fact that prognosis is guarded.

c) Bilateral partial cataracts do not require surgery until the age of 1 to 2 years, but follow up including check up of vision is necessary. If the visual acuity cannot be determined or if the density of cataract seems to impede vision, early surgery is advocated.

d) In Unilateral partial cataract, surgery may be delayed with conservative treatment like mydriasis of the affected eye and patching of the good eye to prevent amblyopia.

e) In partial cataracts where development of vision is satisfactory, surgery may be delayed until 6 to 8 years of age and an IOL is always implanted.

Preferred surgical techniques:

The surgical technique to be adopted to remove the cataract dependents on several factors including age of the child, laterality of cataract, development of vision and type of cataract.

The following procedures are available:

1. Lensectomy with anterior vitrectomy through pars plana approach.
2. Extracapsular Cataract surgery involves anterior capsulorhexis, aspiration of lens matter, posterior capsule capsulorhexis, anterior vitrectomy and IOL implantation.
3. Standard Phaco with intact posterior capsule and PC IOL implantation.

PREOPERATIVE INVESTIGATIONS:

Eye examination: Examination of children below 6 months of age is not difficult and can be examined with the help of an assistant. Most important is to look at pupillary reflex to light and the red reflex with the direct ophthalmoscope and Indirect Ophthalmoscope.

1. Presence pupillary reflex to light: is important in the presence of opaque media due to dense cataract.
2. Examination of Red reflex with direct ophthalmoscope: The opacity shows up as dark shadow in the pupillary area when viewed with + 6 D lens of the ophthalmoscope with pupil fully dilated. It may be difficult to dilate the pupil of an infant and Atropine Drops may cause undue systemic reaction and tachycardia.

3. Examination of the Fundus: The retina should be examined with direct and indirect Ophthalmoscope.

4. Examination of eye movement: Nystagmus if present will cause poor vision, but I have seen children who has 6/12 vision and N8 with Nystagmus after congenital cataract surgery and aphakic correction. Therefore, surgery should be performed in both eyes as soon as possible in children in spite of the presence of Nystagmus.

5. Routine Blood tests: Are necessary for General anesthesia and a child specialist and an anesthesiologist should be consulted.

6. Chest X Ray : P-A view

7. Serology: Blood test for TORCH titer to exclude Rubella, Toxoplasma and CMV is important before planning surgery. Rubella children presents with recurrent and protracted inflammation after cataract surgery. Lensectomy with vitrectomy should be performed on all children with positive reports.

## TECHNIQUES OF SURGERY:

It is not possible to make a generalized recommendation about the procedures to be adopted for pediatric cataract surgery. Several procedures are available to the surgeon who has to apply the procedure judiciously to get optimum visual result. If the anterior vitreous is left behind, it condenses and produces central vitreous opacity obscuring vision in spite of a posterior capsular opening which is made by rhexis or laser. In children below 6 years of age, it is important to remove the anterior vitreous to prevent vitreous opacity and retro lenticular membrane formation.

1. **Lensectomy with anterior vitrectomy**: With the development of Vitreous cutters and incorporating Peristaltic or ventury pumps in the system, Pars Plana Lensectomy is now regarded as standard procedure in children below 2 years of age. These eyeballs are small and the eye is entered through the Pars Plana Micro Vitreoretinal (MVR) blade to introduce a 23 G probe. The pars plana point of entry is 2 mm behind the limbus in less than 1year of age. The point of entry is 2.5 mm in 1-4 year olds and 3 mm in children older than 4 years. The vitrector is introduced through the opening and the center of posterior capsule is opened and aspiration of the lens mater along with anterior vitrectomy is performed. This prevents anterior vitreous condensations and reduces inflammation. The port should be closed with 8/0 Nylon or Vicryl suture.

2. **Anterior Chamber approach for lensectomy** and primary posterior capsular rhexis and anterior vitrectomy :

c) The incision in children is difficult and tricky to perform. Children have thinner and less rigid sclera and consequently, it is difficult to create a self sealing wound. Synthetic, absorbable 10-0 or 8/0 sutures are recommended for closure of the wound. If this is not available, 10/0 Nylon should be used and may be removed at any time after healing has taken place. This requires a second anesthesia and should be delayed as much as possible. If a rigid heparin coated PMMA IOL or a foldable IOL is implanted, a scleral tunnel wound is usually preferred via the superior approach which is easier in children than in adults. This approach allows the wound to be protected by the brow and the Bell's phenomenon in the trauma-prone children and also heals better. Clear Corneal Temporal approach incision may also be used provided that, an acrylic foldable IOL is implanted.

d) **Anterior Capsulorhexis**

**Capsulorhexis using forceps**: Capsulorhexis in children requires special skill because the anterior capsule is elastic and rhexis runaway is common. An intact CCC resists tearing once completed successfully. Because of the increased elasticity of the pediatric anterior capsule, more force is required when pulling on the capsular flap before the tearing begins. CCC in children is done with forceps in all cases. In the beginning, the eye should be filled with good viscoelastics to flatten the anterior capsule. The pressure in the anterior chamber must be higher than the pressure in the lens and vitreous. The Capsulorhexis edge needs to be grasped frequently and begin with a capsulotomy smaller than desired. After completion, the rhexis will enlarge. The tearing force must be directed toward the center of the pupil to control the turning of the CCC edge along a circular path. If the capsule begins to extend peripherally, stop and try from another site. If this fails, conversion to other methods of anterior capsulotomy should be considered.

1.) Mechanized circular anterior Capsulorhexis called vitreorhexis is performed using vitreous cutter. The vitrector tip is placed through a tight fit stab incision made at the limbus using a MVR blade. Irrigation is usually provided with a blunt tip irrigating cannula through a separate stab incision. A cut rate of 150 to 300 cycles per minute is recommended. The cutting port is oriented posteriorly and the center of the anterior capsule is aspirated up into the cutting port to create an initial opening. Any nuclear or cortical material that comes out of capsular bag is aspirated easily without interrupting the capsulectomy technique. The capsular opening is enlarged using the cutter in a gentle circular fashion. This technique can be easily performed in cataract that is white. A smooth, round capsulectomy can be produced, which resists radial tearing. The more elastic the anterior capsule, the smoother the edge of the vitrectorhexis appears. The vitrectorhexis technique works best in young patients in whom the manual CCC is more difficult. The vitrectorhexis is less ideal in an older child because the capsule elasticity begins to approach that of an adult capsule.

2.)   Capsulotomy using high frequency endodiathermy: The Bipolar radio frequency endodiathermy is fitted with a 0.6-mm diameter handpiece and tip designed for anterior capsulectomy. A high frequency modulation (500 kHz) signal is set and a low mean energy is delivered, which minimizes the cutting energy and decreases heat generation. The needle tip is placed in contact with the anterior capsule as the tip is activated by pressing the foot pedal. The surgeon controls the capsulectomy size and shape as the tip is moved along a circular path. Gas bubbles form as the capsule is cut and may cause difficulty in visibility. The procedure is performed under viscoelastic. The capsule edge rolls up slightly, which creates a larger capsulectomy than initially cut with the instrument tip. The Fugo Blade has also been used to perform an anterior capsulectomy in children.

e)   **Aspiration of cortical mater**: The cortical mater is usually soft and can be aspirated easily using the irrigation aspiration handpiece of the phaco machine or using Simco Cannula. This can also be performed using the hand piece of the Vitrectomy apparatus. Whatever means is used to aspirate the cortex, the removal should be as complete as possible. Any cortex left behind will cause subsequent inflammation and early proliferation causing opacity and formation of a Soemmering's ring.

f)   **Primary Posterior Capsulotomy** and anterior vitrectomy: A primary posterior capsulotomy is performed using the vitreous cutter and is advanced to remove part of the anterior vitreous whether an Intraocular lens is implanted or not. In children below the age of 6 years, removing the anterior vitreous reduces complications of formation of after cataract and the need of YAG LASER. In children above 6 years of age, the posterior capsule may be left intact and IOL implanted. They can cooperate better with YAG LASER later on and also a secondary anterior vitrectomy may be performed if required.

g)   **IOL Implantation**: There is no confusion to implant an IOL in children above the age of four years. The power of the lens to be implanted should be either + 1.5 D to +2 D hypermetropic. However, many people advocate keeping them emmetropic for better treatment of amblyopia and the Myopic shift in subsequent years is beneficial.

For Children below 2 years of age, lensectomy with anterior vitrectomy is the procedure of choice. Post operative correction of resultant aphakia is by Glasses or suitable contact lens. Although, lens implant at the age of one year has been performed, this does not prove to contribute to the treatment of amblyopia in a large series.

For the treatment between the ages of two years to four years, the choice is between Intraocular Lens implant or making the child aphakic and wait for further development of the eyeball before a secondary IOL implant is performed, both the procedures are acceptable.

The Power calculation towards a hypermetropic side is advocated. There are several nomograms to follow and it depends on the operating surgeon regarding setting the IOL power to aim for postoperative refraction and treatment of Amblyopia. Many surgeons prefer to make the child hypermetropic between +3 to +1 Diopters depending upon the age of the child. Others prefer to make the child emmetropic which is better for amblyopia treatment and then perform a lens exchange after 8 to 10 years of age. Now piggyback IOL and newer designs of IOL are available to use as a secondary implant without removing the primary IOL. Alternatively, secondary PRK or LASIC can be done to treat resultant Myopia.

3. **Phaco with PC IOL implant**: When cataract surgery is performed in children of 6 years of age and older, primary Phaco surgery with foldable PC IOL is implant is usually performed. Anterior capsulotomy is still difficult than adult cases but can be performed easily using high quality viscoelastics and a good rhexis forceps. The nucleus is soft and can be aspirated or phaco in low power is adequate. The IOL power is either emmetropic or 0.5 D hypermetropic. The posterior capsule can be left intact and these children cooperate well for YAG LASER posterior capsulotomy at a later date. Both scleral tunnel and clear corneal tunnel approach can be adopted for the entry and must be closed with one 8/0 Vicryl or 10/0 Nylon suture.

**POST OPERATIVE CARE**: At the end of surgery, one drop topical antibiotic is installed in the conjunctival sac. Some surgeons also prefer to give a subconjunctival injection of Gentamycin and dexamethasone. Antibiotic ointment and atropine ointment are applied and a patch and shield is applied. During the post operative period, atropine drop once daily, Prednesolone acetate 1% drops 6 times daily for 2 weeks and 4 times daily for 2 weeks and 3 times daily for 2 weeks, antibiotic eye drops 4 times daily for 4 to 6 weeks is given. Refractive correction for resultant refractive error should be given as soon as the wound stabilizes and the sutures are absorbed.

## POST OPERATIVE COMPLICATIONS:

1. Posterior capsular opacification is a major complication of pediatric cataract surgery. Opacification of the anterior hyaloid may occur even if posterior capsulorhexis is performed. This is reduced if posterior capsulorhexis is combined with vitrectomy.

2. Proliferation of lens epithelium usually do not cause visual problem if the central optical axis is not affected but a Soemmering's ring formation may be noted in most cases.

3. Secondary membranes may form across the pupil, particularly if associated chronic uveitis. Thin membranes can be treated with YAG laser but thick membranes may require surgical excision and vitrectomy.

4. Glaucoma eventually develops in about 20% of eyes. IOP should be measured at every visit. Tonopen is usually used, alternatively, Air Puff Tonometer also gives an indication of rise of IOP and if in doubt, an EUA and measurement of IOP with Perkins Applanation tonometer should be performed and appropriate treatment given for secondary glaucoma. Closed angle glaucoma and Secondary open-angle glaucoma may also develop many years after the initial surgery. It is therefore important to monitor the intraocular pressure regularly.

5. Retinal detachment may occur any time after childhood cataract surgery.

**MANAGEMENT OF AMBLYOPIA**: Management of amblyopia is the most important consideration in the post operative years until the child is 12 years of age. Patching of the good eye and working with the bad eye for specific number of hours is the standard treatment. Other forms of pleoptic treatment may also be beneficial. In bilateral cataracts, development of vision is usually good if surgery is undertaken at the appropriate age. In Unilateral cataracts, development of vision depends upon many factors and proper counseling of the parents is of utmost benefit.

## REFERENCES :

1. Koch DD, Kohnen T. Retrospective comparison of techniques to prevent secondary cataract formation after posterior chamber intraocular lens implantation in infants and children. J Cataract Refract Surg. 1997;23:657-663.

2. Vasavada AR, Trivedi RH, Singh R. Necessity of vitrectomy when optic capture is performed in children older than 5 years. J Cataract Refract Surg. 2001;27:1185-1193.

3. Gimbel HV, DeBroff DM. Posterior capsulorhexis with optic capture: Maintaining a clear visual axis after pediatric cataract surgery. *J Cataract Refract Surg.* 1994;20:658-664.

4. Vasavada AR, Trivedi RH. Role of optic capture in congenital and intraocular lens surgery in children. *J Cataract Refract Surg.* 2000;26:824-831.

5. Koch DD, Kohnen T. Retrospective comparison of techniques to prevent secondary cataract formation after posterior chamber intraocular lens implantation in infants and children. *J Cataract Refract Surg.* 1997;23:657-663.

6. Wilson ME. Management of aphakia in childhood. *Focal Points*. American Academy of Ophthalmology. March 1999;17;(1):1-18.

7. Lambert SR, Drack AV. Infantile cataracts. *Surv Ophthalmol.* 1996;40:427-458.

8. Taylor D. The Doyne lecture: Congenital cataract: The history, the nature, and the practice. *Eye.* 1998;12:9-36.

9. Huber C. Increasing myopia in children with intraocular lenses: An experiment in form deprivation myopia. *Eur J Implant Ref Surg.* 1993;5:154-158.

10. Sinskey RM, Stoppel JO, Amin PA. Ocular axial length changes in a pediatric patient with aphakia and pseudophakia. *J Cataract Refract Surg.* 1993;19: 787-788.

11. Vasavada AR, Trivedi RH, Singh R. Necessity of vitrectomy when optic capture is performed in children older than 5 years. *J Cataract Refract Surg.* 2001;27:1185-1193.

12. Choyce DP. Correction of uniocular aphakia by means of anterior chamber acrylic implants. *Trans Ophthalmol Society UK.* 1958;78:459-470.

13. Wilson ME. Anterior capsule management for pediatric intraocular lens implantation. *J Pediatr Ophthalmol Strabismus.* 1999;36:1-6.

14. Kloti R. Anterior high frequency (HF) capsulotomy. Part I: Experimental study. *Klin Monatsbl Augenheilkd.* 1992;2000:507-510.

15. Fugo RJ, Coccio D, McGrann D, Becht L, DelCampo D. The Fugo Blade...the next step after capsulorhexis. Presented at the American Society of Cataract and Refractive Surgery symposium on cataract, IOL and refractive surgery, Congress on Ophthalmic Practice Management, Boston, Massachusetts, May 23, 2001.

16. Vasavada A, Chauhan H. Intraocular lens implantation in infants with congenital cataracts. *J Cataract Refract Surg.* 1994;20:592-598.

17. Parks, MM. Posterior lens capsulectomy during primary cataract surgery in children. *Ophthalmology.* 1983;90:344-345

18. Trivedi R, Vasavada AR, Apple DJ, et al. Cortical cleaving hydrodissection in congenital cataract surgery. Presented at the American Society of Cataract and Refractive Surgery symposium on cataract, IOL and refractive surgery, San Diego, CA, April 29, 2001.

19. Andreo LK, Wilson ME, Apple DJ. Elastic properties and scanning electron microscopic appearance of manual continuous curvilinear capsulorhexis and vitrectorhexis in the animal model of pediatric cataracts. *J Cataract Refract Surg.* 1999;25:534-539.

20. Wilson ME, Bluestein EC, Wang XH, et al. Comparison of mechanized anterior capsulectomy and manual continuous capsulorhexis in pediatric eyes. *J Cataract Refract Surg.* 1994;20:602-606.

# REFRACTIVE CATARACT SURGERY

# CORRECTING ASTIGMATISM WITH LIMBAL RELAXING INCISIONS

# ADVANCED TECHNIQUES IN CATARACT SURGERY

## DR. MEHDI (MATTI) VAZEEN MD

## Chapter 21 A
# REFRACTIVE CATARACT SURGERY

Cataract surgery has become so precise over the past five years that we can now accurately give our patients the desired refractive outcome they wish for.

The goal of refractive cataract surgery is to achieve the desired refractive correction the patient desires. Whether this desire is spectacle independence for distance or for near or both.

In this chapter I shall outline the necessary steps to produce your desired outcome. There are three steps that need to be mastered for consistent results in refractive cataract surgery.

These three steps are:

- Patient selection
- Accurate measurements
- Precise surgery

To achieve the desired results you must perfect these steps.

**Patient selection**

What the patient desires and what you can deliver can sometimes be very far apart. Therefore proper patient selection is very important in the overall process. For example, if a patient has macular degeneration and loss of central vision, obviously they would not benefit from the extra steps of refractive cataract surgery. So we need to make sure that we tell patients honestly what we can deliver to them in terms of final vision.

Select patients obviously with normal eyes, no corneal pathology, no macular pathology and no severe dry eyes or keratitis. Choose patients where the only factors limiting perfect vision (6/6) is refractive error and lens pathology. So when we correct their refractive error and remove their cataracts they achieve emmetropia (6/6) vision.

Ask the patient simple questions, what is it you want? (i.e. distance vision, reading vision, or both.) Ask the patient what is the main difficulty they are having with their vision? (Glare at night, reading small print, and watching TV) Also ask the patient what they do? Do they drive at night? Do they work up close all day? By asking these simple questions you can decide what the patient needs.

**Accurate measurements**

Obviously if time is not taken for accurate measurement and lens selection then all other steps become irrelevant. What do you need for accurate measurement? To do this you need well trained staff. (Remember that garbage measurements produce garbage results) What are the components of accurate IOL calculations (from Warren Hill) Dr. Hill has spent a lifetime accurately perfecting and improving IOL power calculation and his papers are great for further reading for IOL power calculations.

1.) **Pre-operative keratometry measurement**
   a. manual keratometry reading (rarely done now and is not as accurate as computers)
   b. IOL master or other device reading "K"
   c. topography "K" measurements (Orbscan or Ziess units)

I personally obtain my keratometry measurements from the IOL master or topography K readings.

If the patient is paying extra for perfect vision we also perform a macular OCT to rule out any other pathology that may affect our surgical outcome.

2.) **Measurement of axial length. There are various devices that measure the axial length.**
   a). Applanation ultrasound biometry (this is the least accurate system and is dependent on well trained staff for accurate results.)
   b). Immersion ultrasound biometry
   c). Optical biometry.
      1. Zeiss IOL Master System
      2. Haag Streit System

Optical biometry is very accurate and really is the standard of care in the United States. Optical biometry is accurate for all eyes however it is even better than ultrasound in extremely myopic or hyperopic eyes.

**IOL power calculation formula:**

1.) Which IOL power formula should I use?
   a.) Holladay II (very accurate for very myopic or hyperopic eyes)
   b.) Hoffer Q
   c.) SRK/ T I or SRK/T II
   d.) There are more options to choose so pick the one that gives you the best results.
   e.) Final step is each surgeon due to his own surgical technique will need his own surgeon factor to add to the accuracy of these measurements.

**Precise Surgery**

"In cataract surgery every step is built upon the preceding step."

After twenty thousand surgeries I cannot stress how important and yet obvious the above statement is. However, beginning surgeons always seem to get stuck at a surgical step and wonder why. For example if you do not do a good hydrodissection you cannot rotate the lens well, and then run into trouble during your phaco and aspiration of cortex stage.

"This is millimeter surgery". Once again a very obvious statement, but to achieve reproducible refractive outcomes we must have reproducible technique. The technique should not deviate more than a few millimeters. For example, to achieve accurate refractive outcome your capsulorhexis must not deviate more than 1-2 mm in diameter from case to case. So it should always have a diameter between 5 mm to 6.5 mm.

**Refractive cataract techniques for precise surgery**

In this section I will review the necessary surgical steps needed to achieve reproducible refractive cataract surgery.

1.) Correction of the patients' astigmatism, either with limbal relaxing incisions or toric intraocular lenses.

2.) Creation of incision

3.) Creation of Capsulorhexis

4.) Safe phaco emulsification

5.) Lens implantation

Mastering each of these five steps is necessary in achieving excellent refractive results.

In the next chapter I shall discuss correcting astigmatism and the nomograms needed for (LRI). As this is a whole chapter in itself.

Step 1. Treating the patient's astigmatism is obviously needed in achieving our refractive goals.

Step 2. When performing cataract surgery we need to make sure that our incision does not change in size or position from case to case, as a large incision ≥ 3mm or superior temporal or inferior temporal incision can affect our refractive outcome by greater than 0.6 D (warren hill studied and stressed the importance of this). So an ideal incision should be placed always within one o'clock hour of the surgeon's preference. The incision should also have an opening between 2 and 3mm. now as long as these two parameters do not change within thirty five cases a surgeon factor can be developed to compensate for any refractive errors these steps produce.

Step 3. Studies have shown that too large of a capsulorhexis size ≥ 6mm or too small in size ≤ 5mm can increase inaccuracy by changing the final resting place of the lens. A large capsulorhexis will leave the lens vaulted back toward the macula resulting in greater hyperopia, while a small capsulorhexis will result in the lens vaulting forward with a more myopic result. So the surgeon must practice producing a 5mm-6mm capsulorhexis that covers the optic by 1mm-2mm all the way around for best refractive results.

Step 4. Safe phacoemulsification implies that the lens is removed without any damage to the zonular system causing weakness and lens shift and therefore refractive change.

Step 5. Lens placement into the bag. Once again although this is a simple step, if not performed properly can affect the refractive outcome. So proper placement of the lens requires it be placed in the capsular bag with the optic surrounded by 0.5mm to 1mm of the capsule, that the lens is flush against the posterior capsule, all the viscoelastic underneath the lens is removed and that the lens is not tilted in any way.

**In summary: In my practice we are achieving less then ± 0.6 D of refractive error in over 92% of our patients after cataract surgery.**

This high level is achieved by following the steps outlined above.

1.) proper patient selection
2.) accurate measurements
3.) precise reproducible surgery

Over time (20,000 surgeries and counting) if you as a surgeon monitor every step of the procedure you can then identify where your results are deviating and need to be adjusted. Therefore sticking to a technique that does not change more than a few millimeters for each case, we can then figure out where along the path we need to make adjustments for better surgical results.

**References:**

1. Warren E. Hill, MD FACS East Valley Ophthalmology Mesa, Arizona USA
2. Kim SJ, Bressler NM: optical coherence tomography and cataract surgery. Curr opin Ophthalmol 20:464, 2009
3. Tally-Rostoy A: patient-centered care and refractive cataract surgery. Curr opin ophthalmol 19:5, 2008
4. Aimsbury EC, Miller KM: correction if astigmatism at the time of cataract surgery. Curr opin ophthalmol 20:52
5. Cionne RJ et al: clinical outcomes and functional visual performance: comparison of the ReStor apodized diffractive intraocular lens to a monofocal control. Br J ophthalmol 93:1215, 2009
6. Langenbucher A et al: Toric intraocular lenses--- Theory, Matrix calculations, and clinical practice. J refract surg 25:611, 2009
7. Maxwell WA, et al: Performance of presbyopia- correcting intraocular lenses in distance optical bench test. J cataract refract surg 35:166 2009
8. Pepose JS: Maximizing satisfaction with presbyopia- correcting intraocular lenses: the missing links, Am J ophthalmol 146:641, 2008

# Chapter 21 B

# CORRECTING ASTIGMATISM IN CATARACT SURGERY

If we desire to implant premium lenses (multifocal) or want to provide patients with spectacle independence, we must address astigmatism correction at the time of cataract surgery.

In this chapter I shall discuss gathering data, nomograms to use and surgical technique for correction of astigmatism. I shall also discuss pearls and pitfalls of each of these sections.

To be successful and accurate in correcting astigmatism in cataract surgery you have to commit totally to the process.

1.) All the right equipment must be in place
2.) All the staff must be properly trained and committed to correction of astigmatism

In my specialty practice I perform over one hundred cataract surgeries a month. The whole practice is committed to treating all patients with astigmatism greater than +0.50 D. 90% of post cataract patients have better than 20/25 uncorrected vision.

**There are three main steps in the surgical correction of astigmatism.**

1.) Gathering data
2.) Nomogram use
3.) Surgical technique

**Gathering data**

To achieve accurate astigmatic correction we must have reliable data to guide us in proper location and degree of the incision.

I use three parameters in selecting the axis and the amount of astigmatism I will be correcting.

1.) Refraction in (+) cylinder. (I sometimes use wavefront data)
2.) K reading (manual or off IOL master)
3.) Topography

Collection of data: this should be posted above patients head.

- Manifest refraction
- Keratometry measurements
- Corneal topography

If all three of these parameters match I am very aggressive in correcting all the astigmatism. If only 2/3 out of three match with the same axis (if the two are topography and K's). If topography and K's axis are the opposite or not the same abort, do nothing. You can explain to the patient at the pre-op if they are not a good candidate for correction of astigmatism.

**Nomograms to use**

There are plenty of various different nomograms out there. If you feel comfortable and are getting great results from them, go with any of these or you can prepare your own nomogram. The validity of any of these nomograms is in the results they produce for you, weighing against possible complications.

**The described nomograms are:**

1. **Louis D Nichamin MD – Laurel Eye Clinic PA**
2. **Dr. Gills LRI nomograms**
3. **Donnenfield Nomogram – "DONO"**
4. **Kevin Miller MD LRI Nomogram**
5. **My Nomogram**

You can get any of these nomograms from the original articles by these surgeons. I shall describe the nomogram that I follow.

**My Nomogram**

I tried to keep it simple. I wanted my worst case scenario to be zero irregular astigmatism. Axis determination was important, but did not have to be dead on to correct greater than +1.50 D. In these cases we have the better option of choosing a Toric Intraocular lens.

**Nomogram that I use :**

**Five different parameters**

1.) +0.50 D to+1.00 D
2.) +1.00 D to +1.50 D
3.) +1.50 D to +2.00 D
4.) +2.00 D to +2.50 D
5.) +2.50 D and Greater

**1. Correcting for + 0.50 to +1.00 D :**

The incision is at the Limbus, it should be 120 degree arc as follows :

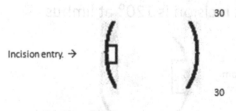

## Correcting for +0.50D to +1.00D.

### The incision should be 120° ARC

Incision entry. →   30

30

### At the limbus.

## 2. Correcting for +1.00 to +1.50 D

The incision should be 1-2 mm from the Limbus 120 Degree arc.

### Correcting for +1.00D to +1.50D.

#### The incision should be 120° arc.

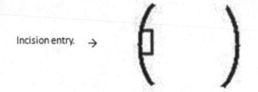

Incision entry. →

### 1-2mm from the limbus.    ↑

## 3. Correcting for + 1.50 to +2.00 D

The first incision should be 1 mm from the limbus 120 degrees radius. The second incision should be 2 mm inside the limbus a length of 45 degree ark at the steep axis.

### Correcting for +1.50D to +2.00D

#### The first incision is 120° at limbus.

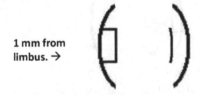

1 mm from
limbus. →

#### The second incision is 2mm inside the limbus at length of 45° ARC. (steep axis of astigmatism)

## 4. Correcting for +2.00 to + 2.50 :

The first incision should be 1 mm from the limbus and 120 degrees arc. The second incision should be 3 mm inside the limbus at steep axis of astigmatism with length of 45 degree arc. Caution is to be followed to remain outside the optical zone.

# Correcting for +2.00D to +2.50D

The first incision is 120° at limbus.

1 mm from limbus. →

The second incision is 3mm inside limbus at steep axis of astigmatism with length of 45° arc. (Stay out of the optical zone.)

## 5. Correcting + 2.50 D and Grater:

The first incision should be 1 mm from the limbus and 120 degrees arc. The second incision should be 4 mm inside the limbus at the steep axis with a length 45 degree arc out side the optical zone.

# Correcting for +2.50D and Greater

The first incision is 120° at limbus.

1 mm from limbus. →

The second incision is 4mm inside limbus at steep axis of astigmatism with length of 45° arc. (Stay out of the optical zone.)

**Nomograms with two paired incisions allows for greater margin of error.**

If your axis is off by five degrees or ten degrees, the second large limbal relaxing incision allows for the prevention of irregular astigmatism. This can be significant if your astigmatism is greater than +1.50 D. The correct <u>axis</u> becomes very important. Also there is less regression noted over time. The arc length of astigmatism correction described in my nomogram is 120 degrees, but an arc length of 90 degree produces the same result and this should be followed.

## Diamond Knife

There are a lot of various astigmatism keratome knives that can be used for your incision. There are adjustable knives where the depth can be adjusted at various microns. I personally use a guarded diamond knife set at 550 μm. This will be at a depth of 80-90% peripheral cornea with a very low chance of perforation since it is guarded at 550 μm and 97% of corneal depth is greater than 600μm in the periphery.

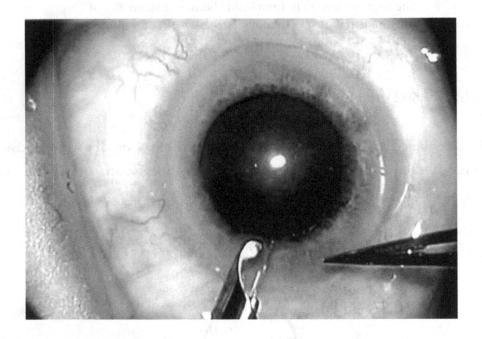

(Fig. 37 : Guarded Diamond blade set at 550 μm)

**Surgical Technique:**

- Use blade set at 550 µm.
- Divide the cornea into four 90 degree zones.
- When you are starting out you should mark the axis.
- Verify the amount of correction with patients refractions, K's, and topography above the patients head
- Ease in to correct steep axis of 90 degrees instead of steep axis of 180 degrees.
- Do cuts before entering the eye.
- Place viscoat over any small bleeders.

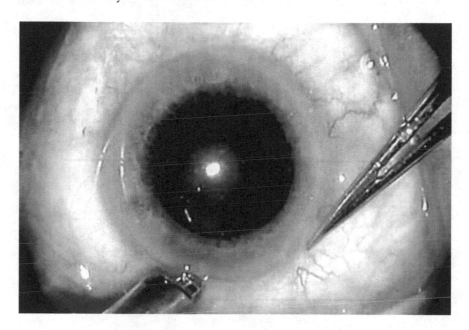

(Fig 38 : LRI with guarded diamond knife)

**Title #1**

I.D. # 25674 refraction prior to surgery:

| O.D. | O.S. |
|------|------|
| -2.50 +1.75×015 | -2.75+1.75×001 |
| K's 0.71@021 | K's 0.94@161 |

Post-op refraction:

Plano Sphere                        Plano sphere

Visual acuity post-op uncorrected OD: 20/20 OS : 20/20

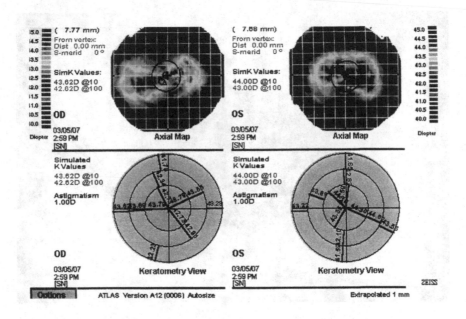

Fig. 39. Topography of patient 1

**Title #2**

I.D. # 10165 refraction prior to surgery:

| O.D. | O.S. |
|---|---|
| -1.75+1.50×167 | -1.00+1.50×175 |
| K's 1.73@001 | K's 1.63@002 |
| Post-op refraction: | |
| -0.50+0.25×115 | Plano sphere |
| Visual acuity post-op uncorrected: | |
| 20/20 | 20/20 |

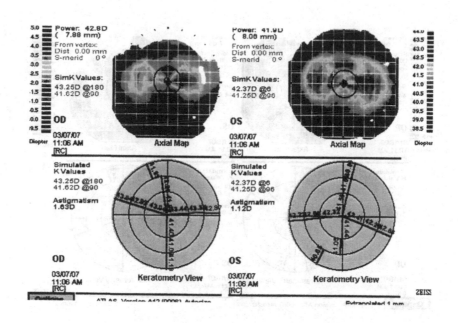

Fig.40 Topography of patient II

**Title #3**

I.D. # 25306 refraction prior to surgery:

O.D. O.S.

-4.00+0.75×055                    -5.25+0.25×110

K's 1.34@089                       K's 0.98@084

Post-op refraction:

Plano Sphere                       -0.25 Sph

Visual acuity uncorrected:

20/20                              20/20

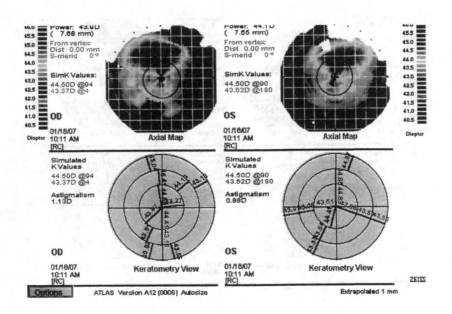

Fig. 41 : Topography of patient III

## Potential problems

- Infection
- Weakening of the globe
- Perforation
- Decreased corneal sensation
- Induced irregular astigmatism
- Misalignment/ axis shift
- Wound gape and discomfort
- Operating upon the wrong axis!

*Reprinted with permission from gills J, ed, A complete surgical guide for correcting astigmatism: an ophthalmic manifesto. Thorofare, NJ: Slack, Inc; 2003*

If you perform LRI's you need to tell the patient they may have some foreign body sensations over the next 3-4 weeks. Most patients are happy due to the reduction of astigmatism. Even a 50% reduction in astigmatism can reduce aberrations significantly. In greater than 2 D of astigmatism you will have over correction.

# Chapter 22
# SPECIALITY INTRAOCULAR LENSES

Several Specialty Intraocular Lenses are available and many are forthcoming. Knowledge about these advancements and options are necessary for a cataract surgeon whether or not these products are available to the surgeon.

1. Multifocal Intraocular Lenses: Several types of multifocal intraocular lenses are available and the mode of action depends upon the design of the platform the individual company uses. These lenses are designed to offer good visual acuity at distance and at near. Full knowledge about calculation of power and centration of these lenses is important before one can implant these lenses. The company that produces the lens usually offers full instructions and assists in power calculation and other technical support. Multifocal lens cannot be implanted if the preexisting astigmatism is more than +/- 1.5 Dioptres of corneal astigmatism unless this is also corrected by LRI or other methods.

2. Toric Intraocular Lenses : Toric Intraocular lenses correct existing corneal astigmatism. The monofocal Toric lenses correct distance power including the astigmatism, so that the patient do not require glasses postoperatively to correct astigmatism. The power calculation and axis cylinder calculations has to be exact and the manufacturing company gives power calculators to chose the exact lens to be implanted.

3. Toric –Multifocal Intraocular lenses: Toric and multifocal combination is available and is offered by some companies which correct both astigmatism and accommodation.

4. Pseudophakic Supplementary Introcular Lenses: Phacoemulsification and IOL implantation is designed to correct refractive power up to 0.5 Diopter accuracy. In the event that, while performing phaco surgery, a big after refraction happens to be the outcome, the surgeons have a choice to implant a supplementary intraocular lens to correct the resulting refractive power. One such patented lens is SulcoFlex pseudophakic supplementary IOL from Rayner IOL company, of Hove, UK.

5. New designs of intraocular lenses are devised by different companies to make it as stable as possible inside the bag so that Multifocal and Toric Multifocal lenses can be centered to give the expected refractive outcome.

6. Future Intraocular Lenses: In the future, new lens models and materials are under investigation which will give customized power determination and accommodation. Research is underway and the days are not far away when we will have lenses which are custom made and will give better quality of vision than the normal human lens in the eye.

# Chapter 23

# LASER ASSISTED CATARACT SURGERY: FEMTOSECOND LASER

New techniques and instruments and equipments continue to evolve in the field of cataract surgery. Research into the field of Lasers and Phaco machines and Lens designs has brought about revolutionary developments and will continue to bring changes in the field of cataract surgery. It is beyond the scope of this book to describe all the new developments and research that is being performed in this field. The discussion on Femtosecond Laser is necessary because the Phaco Surgeons will eventually confront with this technology sooner or later.

Femtosecond Laser is a Passive Mode Locking Laser system that emits ultra short optical pulses in ultrafast time scale in the domain of Femtosecond where 1 Fs = 10x-15 second. In the modern machines, the surgeon first makes a precise incision plan with the help of 3-D image of the eye with integrated OCT into the machine which gives high accuracy to the incision site, depth and length in all planes. The Femtosecond Laser can be utilized to perform the following tasks in cataract surgery: 1) Clear Corneal Incisions 2) Capsulorhexis which is exact CCC in measurement and position, 3) Laser Cutting and softening of the Nucleus, 4) Astigmatism correction by Limbal Relaxing incisions

Without going into the technical details, the procedure requires two equipments, the Femtosecond Laser equipment and a Phacoemulsification machine.

**DOCKING AND CORNEAL INCISION**

First the patient is oriented with the LASER machine which requires a soft contact lens to be fitted to the cornea with enough suction to Applanate the cornea and make it ready for the Laser to work. The OCT image is created for accurate incision and the LASER creates the clear corneal incision. The docking system causes some increase of intraocular pressure. The parasentesis and limbal relaxing incisions can also be planned at the same time using the OCT as a guide to an accurate depth.

## CAPSULOTOMY:

Manually performed CCC is important to be of correct size and cent

ration. When performed by the LASER, the CCC can be accurately planned using the OCT as a guide to prepare a well centered and round Rhexis of appropriate size.

## SOFTENING OF THE NUCLEUS

For phacoemulsification to work, the nucleus needs to be broken to small bite size pieces which are performed by Cracking of the nucleus. The nucleus can be softened to crack easily using the LASER system. The nucleus is marked and the depth of the crack is ascertained and the laser will cut into the correct depth to create specified number of nuclear pieces which can then be emulsified using the standard phacoemulsification systems.

## TRANSFERING THE PATIENT TO THE PHACO MACHINE:

After the initial preparation with the LASER, the patient is then transferred to the Phaco Machine for phacoemulsification and removal of the nucleus, removal of the cortical mater and implantation of the Intraocular Lens in the bag.

## LASER CATARACT SURGERY SYSTEMS PRESENTLY AVAILABLE ARE:

1. **LenSx.** The LenSx (Alcon) is Femtosecond laser system patented by ALCON and is FDA approved for cataract surgery. The machine is capable to perform three aspects of cataract surgery: Creating the anterior capsulotomy, fragmenting the cataract and making laser incisions for Clear Corneal Incision.
2. **LensAR.** The latest LensAR Laser System (LensAR, Inc.) is approved by FDA for anterior capsulotomy and lens fragmentation and corneal incisions.
3. **Catalys.** The Catalys Precision Laser System (OptiMedica) is approved for capsulotomy and lens fragmentation.
4. **Victus.** The Victus Femtosecond Laser Platform (Technolas Perfect Vision with Bausch + Lomb). The Victus is a multiple-use femtosecond laser system that can perform anterior capsulotomy during cataract surgery; corneal flap creation during LASIK surgery or other treatment requiring initial lamellar resection and corneal incisions.

Several other Femtosecond Laser systems are in the process of trial for the purpose of Cataract surgery and creation of flap in LASIC surgery.

sSUMMARY :

Whatever Laser system is used, all perform the same objective of precisely cutting the tissues. Since Cataract surgery is a surgery of precision, the Laser system has lots of potential in this field and it is possible that in the coming years, Femtosecond Lasers will make a revolution to the way we perform cataract surgery today. Present outlook of the procedure shows that it is safe for certain procedures of the surgical steps. Further research and evaluation will tell us whether this new procedure will be beneficial to the patients and the cost effectiveness of the procedure.

**References :**

1. Friedman NJ, Palanker DV, Schuele G, Andersen D, Marcellino G, Seibel BS, et al. Femtosecond laser capsulotomy. J Cataract Refract Surg. 2011;37:1189–98.
2. Murphy C, Tuft SJ, Minassian DC. Refractive error and visual outcome after cataract extraction. J Cataract Refract Surg. 2002;28:62–6
3. Palanker DV, Blumenkranz MS, Andersen D, Wiltberger M, Marcellino G, Gooding P, et al. Femtosecond laser-assisted cataract surgery with integrated optical coherence tomography. Sci Transl Med. 2010;2:58
4. Cekic O, Batman C. The relationship between capsulorhexis size and anterior chamber depth relation. Ophthalmic Surg Lasers. 1999;30:185–90
5. He L, Sheehy K, Culbertson W. Femtosecond laser-assisted cataract surgery. Curr Opin Ophthalmol. 2011;22:43–52.
6. Kránitz K, Takacs A, Mihaltz K, Kovacs I, Knorz MC, Nagy ZZ. Femtosecond laser capsulotomy and manual continuous curvilinear capsulorrhexis parameters and their effects on intraocular lens centration. J Refract Surg. 2011:1–6.

# INDEX

## WESTERN NEVADA SURGICAL CENTER, INC.
## PATIENT SAFETY CHECKLIST

**Patient Name:**

| PRE-PROCEDURE | SIGN-IN | TIME OUT | SIGN-OUT |
|---|---|---|---|
| Pre-Op | Before Induction of Anesthesia and Incision | Before Incision | Before the Patient leaves the Operating Room |
| **Patient/patient representative actively confirms with RN:** | **RN, Anesthesia Care Provider and Scrub Tech confirm:** | **Initiated by Circulator** All other activities to be suspended (unless a life threatening emergency) | **RN Confirms:** |
| Identity: ☐Yes | Procedure, Procedure Site and consent(s): ☐ Yes | Introduction of team members: ☐ Yes | Name of operative procedure Completion of sponge, sharp and Instrument counts: ☐ Yes ☐ N/A |
| Procedure/procedure site: ☐ Yes | Site Marked: ☐ Yes by person performing the procedure | Confirmation of the following: Identity, procedure, incision site, Consent(s) ☐ Yes | |
| Consent(s): ☐ Yes | | | Specimens identified and labeled: ☐ Yes ☐ N/A |
| Site Marked: ☐ Yes ☐ N/A by person performing procedure | Patient Allergies: ☐ Yes ☐ N/A | Site is marked and visible: ☐ Yes ☐ N/A | Any equipment problems to be addressed? ☐ Yes ☐ No |
| **RN Confirms presence of:** | Difficult airway or aspiration risk? ☐ No | Relevant images properly labeled and displayed: ☐ Yes ☐ N/A | Patient Stable for transfer to PACU ☐ Yes |
| History and Physical: ☐ Yes | ☐ Yes (preparation confirmed) | Any equipment concerns? ☐ Yes ☐ No | **To all team members:** What are the key concerns for recovery and management of this pt? |
| Pre-anesthesia Assessment: ☐Yes | **Anesthesia Provider:** Anesthesia Safety Check Completed: ☐ Yes | **Anticipated Critical Events:** **Surgeon:** States the following: ☐ Critical or non-routine steps | Circulator reports to post-op RN all pertinent information relevant to a discharge without complications |
| Any special equipment, devices, Implants: ☐ Yes ☐ No | **Anesthesia Provider:** ☐ Antibiotic prophylaxis within one hour before incision: ☐ Yes ☐ No ☐ Additional concerns? | ☐ Case duration | **PACU:** ☐ Patient monitored for stable vital signs ☐ Patient transferred to 2nd stage after documentation of stable vital signs |
| | Briefing: All members of the team have discussed care plan and addressed concerns: ☐ Yes | **Scrub and Circulating Nurse:** ☐ Sterilization indicators have been confirmed (printout verified) ☐ Additional concerns? | ☐ Patient meets discharge criteria and all discharge instructions given by RN and understood by patient |
| Pre-Op RN:_____ | Circulator:_____ | | Post-Op RN:_____ |

294